Medical Statistics Made Easy

Medical Statistics
Made Easy

Fiona Broughton Pipkin M.A., D.Phil.

Senior Lecturer in Reproductive Physiology,
University of Nottingham

CHURCHILL LIVINGSTONE
EDINBURGH LONDON MELBOURNE AND NEW YORK 1984

CHURCHILL LIVINGSTONE
Medical Division of Longman Group UK Limited

Distributed in the United States of America by
Churchill Livingstone Inc., 1560 Broadway, New York,
N.Y. 10036, and by associated companies, branches
and representatives throughout the world.

First published 1984
  Reprinted 1986

ISBN 0 443 02888 5

British Library Cataloguing in Publication Data

Pipkin, Fiona Broughton
  Medical statistics made easy.
  1. Medical statistics
  I. Title
  519.5'02461   RA409

Produced by Longman Singapore Publishers Pte Ltd
Printed in Singapore

Preface

This small book arose from a series of lectures on basic statistics given to candidates working for the Diploma and Membership of the Royal College of Obstetricians and Gynaecologists. A frequent plea was 'Why isn't there a book which explains it like that?' and referral to the texts suggested for further reading at the end of this book did not seem to answer the question. Hence *Medical Statistics Made Easy*.

It has been written as simply as possible, with worked examples for every concept introduced. There are in addition questions at the end of Chapters 2–7 for the reader to attempt, which also have worked answers.

An important feature of the book is the summary at the end of each of Chapters 2–7 which, it is hoped, will be useful as general reminders for reference, and for revision. There is also a brief summary of all equations used, at the end of the book. *Please* do not attempt to use only these summaries without first reading the book, which tries to explain *why* you do *what* you do.

I am grateful to the Literary Executor of the late Sir Ronald A. Fisher FRS, to Dr Frank Yates FRS and to Longman Group Ltd, London for permission to reprint Tables I, III, IV, V and VI from their book *Statistical Tables for Biological, Agricultural and Medical Research* (6th Edition, 1974). I am also grateful to Dr A.A. Rimm and to Appleton-Century-Crofts, New York, for permission to reprint Appendices 2, 9, 10, 11 and 12 from the book *Basic Biostatistics in Medicine and Epidemiology* (1980).

I am most grateful to my friends and colleagues who have read and criticised the manuscript and made many helpful suggestions. I am also deeply indebted to Catherine Greasley and Lynne Broughton, who tackled the typing with their usual courage and cheerfulness, even in the face of a liberal scattering of the Greek alphabet.

Nottingham, 1984   F.B.P.

Contents

Chapter 1: Some basic concepts   1

    Scales of measurement
    Samples
    Hypotheses
    Probability
    Type I and Type II error
    Incidence and prevalence
    Crude and standardized rates

Chapter 2: Normal or Gaussian distribution   9

    Basic description
    Variance and standard deviation
    Outliers
    Use of tables of z
    Cut-off points
    Classification
    Standard errors
    Confidence intervals
    Coefficient of variation
    Skewed distribution
    Summary of Chapter 2
    Questions for Chapter 2

Chapter 3: Other distributions   32

    The binomial distribution
    The chi-squared (χ^2) distribution
    χ^2 and goodness of fit
    Summary of Chapter 3
    Questions for Chapter 3

Chapter 4: Simple significance tests   46

    Ranking tests
    χ^2 again
    2×2 contingency tables
    Fisher's exact test
    Wilcoxon's signed rank test
    Wilcoxon's ranking test for unpaired
        data (Mann-Whitney test)
    Summary of Chapter 4
    Questions for Chapter 4

Chapter 5: More simple significance tests 66

Large samples ($n > 30$)
The comparison of two percentages
Small samples (either or both $n \leqslant 30$)
Degrees of freedom in 't' tests
Unpaired samples when the F test is significant
One and two-tailed tests
Summary of Chapter 5
Questions for Chapter 5

Chapter 6: A brief introduction to the analysis of variance 85

Summary of Chapter 6
Questions for Chapter 6

Chapter 7: Correlation and regression 91

χ^2 yet again
Spearman's rank correlation coefficient
Correlation
Linear regression analysis
Extrapolation
Summary of Chapter 7
Questions for Chapter 7

Chapter 8: Pitfalls for the unwary 106

Suggested further reading 109

Glossary of symbols 110

Summary guide to equations 112

Appendices 1–9 122

Index 135

1

Some basic concepts

Les statistiques sont comme les bikinis; elles donnent une idée
mais cachent l'essentiel

Anon

From the time when a baby first realises that it has two arms, two legs
and one head, it is capable of making assessments of number. It will
use such assessments, both consciously and unconsciously, for the
rest of its life. The art and science of statistics is no more than an
extension of this ability, being concerned with the collection and
organisation of data, and with its subsequent evaluation.

This brief introduction is not designed as, or intended to be, a
comprehensive statistical textbook. Numerous such books are already available, of varying degrees of sophistication. This is an
attempt to explain, as simply as possible, some of the basic ideas
underlying commonly used statistics, in the hope that if the principles
are understood, the practice becomes that much easier.

Scales of measurement

Since statistics are concerned with measurements, it is important to
realise that there are more ways of measuring things than by simply
applying a numerical value to them. For example, eye colour cannot
be given a direct numerical value in the same way that height can. In
this instance, eye colour could be reported on a _nominal_ (naming)
scale, such as:

Eye colour: blue, grey, green, brown, black

Another example of a nominal scale would be:

Country of origin: England, Ireland, Scotland, Wales

These are examples of _non-parametric_ measurements to which _no_
numerical value can be assigned.

Another scale of measurement is the _ordinal_ (ordering) scale.
Suppose that you were asked to judge a 'beautiful baby' contest. You

cannot assign a direct numerical value to the babies, but you will finally arrive at a decision, such as:

1st: Baby Brown   2nd: Baby Smith   3rd: Baby Jones

In this example you have put them *in order* of (personal) preference. Another way of saying this is that you have *ranked* them.

A further example of an ordinal scale is that of the reporting of examination results. In this instance actual numerical values may be available, but it may be considered more desirable to report them simply in order. So if three candidates Jim Jones, Susan Smith and Bill Brown had actual marks of 53, 76 and 68% respectively, on an ordinal scale they would be placed as:

1st: Susan Smith   2nd: Bill Brown   3rd: Jim Jones

This is an example of the transformation of parametric data to a non-parametric scale. Remember that you now have no information about *how much* better Susan Smith's marks were than Bill Brown's, only that they *were* better.

The actual examination marks suggested above come from a further scale of measurement, the *interval* scale. This is used whenever it is possible to measure a variable so that the difference between any two neighbouring points on the scale of measurement is identical. So, for the scale:

1, 2, 3, 4, 5, 6, 7

there is one unit of difference between 1 and 2, one unit difference between 2 and 3, one unit difference between 6 and 7 and so on. Height, weight, age, serum electrolyte concentrations and blood pressures are all routinely reported on an interval scale. This is *parametric* data.

Remember that if you know, for example, the weights of a group of patients, you can always convert this parametric data to non-parametric by ranking in an ordinal scale (see above). There are times when it is useful to be able to do this.

Since a considerable proportion of statistics is concerned with data measured on an interval scale, it is useful to understand a few basic concepts of numerical measurement. For instance, what exactly is an accurate measurement? A measurement is said to be *accurate* if it matches exactly an accepted standard.

e.g. A thermometer which read 103°C for pure water boiling at sea level and 760 mmHg barometric pressure would be *in*accurate, since it should read 100°C.

Accuracy is often confused with precision but they are quite different. A *precise* measurement is one made in very small units.

e.g. A patient weighed on a balance which measured to the nearest 100 gm, rather than the nearest kilogram, has been weighed with ten times more precision. It is therefore possible for a measurement to be both precise and inaccurate.

A measurement is said to be *reliable* if it can be repeated with minimal variation.

e.g. The height of an adult will be a reliable measurement. Measurement of casual blood pressure is, however, a very *un*reliable measurement.

A *valid* measurement is one which gives genuine information about what is being measured.

e.g. The measurement of 24 h urinary oestrogen concentration will be *in*valid in a patient taking ampicillin.

Samples
Statistics are usually used to describe characteristics of *populations* by extrapolation from *samples*. It is therefore important to ensure that any sample is as representative as possible of the population from which it is drawn. There are some logical steps which can be taken. The sample *size,* usually expressed as n (number), should, in general terms, be as large as possible. Obviously, if one is considering a population of 1000 individuals, a sample of 100 is logically likely to be more representative than one of 10. This is especially true if one is looking for, for example, small changes in response to treatment, or at conditions which are present only rarely in the population. A trained statistician should be consulted early in the planning stages of a project, to give advice on suitable sample size for the problem which you are considering.

Known potential sources of *bias* in sampling should be avoided. Thus if one wished to assess the incidence of a blood alcohol concentration in excess of 80 mg.dl^{-1} in the population *as a whole*, one would not sample a crowd at a race-meeting. What is required is a *random* sample, in which every member of the population has an equal chance of selection. Again, statisticians are happy to give advice concerning random sampling techniques.

Hypotheses
Whenever one is assessing whether an individual (abnormal) value is

likely to have come from a normal population, or whether treatment with a new drug is having a significantly better effect than with an old, or whether mortality rates from bronchial carcinoma are changing, one is, whether consciously or otherwise, testing a hypothesis. Hypotheses by their nature cannot be proved, but they can be accepted or rejected on the basis of available evidence. By convention, statistical hypotheses are given the form that 'The individual value will have come from the general population (i.e. that it is *not* different)', that 'Treatment with the new drug is *not* significantly better than treatment with the old,' that 'Mortality rates from bronchial carcinoma are *not* changing'. These are all known as *Null Hypotheses,* and can be symbolically summarised as:

$$H_0: f_{ob} = f_{ex} \text{ or } H_0: f_{ob} - f_{ex} = 0$$

which is shorthand for:

'The null hypothesis (H_0) states that the observed frequency of an event $(f_{ob}$; the proportion of times when it occurs) will not differ from that expected (f_{ex}) either from theoretical reasoning or previous evidence'.

This will be illustrated more fully in the first few worked examples in the next chapter.

Probability

The concept of probability is an important one in relation both to descriptive and comparative statistics. It is also, however, a concept with which many people initially find difficulty.

Probabilities are conventionally expressed as proportions. A cast-iron certainty, such as the proposition that:

'All men will die'

can be given a probability of 100%, usually expressed as:

$$P = 1.0$$

where P stands for probability.

All other probabilities are measured by comparison with this standard of unity. For example, if there is one chance in twenty that something will happen, this is equivalent to 5 chances in 100, or 5%. This is written as:

$$P = 0.05$$

Similarly, 1 chance in $\quad 100 = 1.0\%, \quad P = 0.01$
and $\qquad$ 1 chance in $\quad 500 = 0.2\%, \quad P = 0.002$
and $\qquad$ 1 chance in $1000 = 0.1\%, \quad P = 0.001$

It is conventional to consider that if there has been shown to be less than one chance in twenty of the observed effect having arisen if the Null Hypothesis is valid then the effect is *statistically significant*. This is an arbitrary, but almost universally-used, cut-off point. The phrase 'statistically highly significant' is usually reserved for those instances where there is less than one chance in one thousand of the observed effect arising, but this usage varies somewhat from author to author.

Another point to remember is the logical one of the *meaning* of probability. If a fair die is thrown, it can be said that the probability of throwing a 6 is 1/6 or $P = 0.166$. However, as anyone who has done it knows, this does *not* mean that exactly one throw out of every six will produce a 6. If a die is thrown 60 times, it is *likely* that a 6 will be thrown 10 times. Even throwing a die 600 times may not give *exactly* 100 6s.

A further point to remember is this. Imagine a treatment for cancer which has a 90% success rate, but the remaining 10% die. If two patients come to you for treatment, what is the probability that one will die?

The probability of either patient dying is 0.1 (1/10) and the probability of either *not* dying is therefore 0.9 (9/10). The probability of both recovering is then $(0.9 \times 0.9 =) 0.81$ while the probability of both dying is $(0.1 \times 0.1 =) 0.01$. The balance of probability is thus $[1 - (0.81 + 0.01)] = 0.18$ (rather less than one in five) that one will die. This, while fairly straightforward when one thinks about it, is not the answer that immediately springs to mind. Be careful when interpreting this kind of information!

Finally, but possibly most importantly, do remember that statistical and biological significance are *not* necessarily the same thing. A new drug may kill statistically-significantly more micro-organisms *in vitro* than an older one but if *in vivo* they can still replicate to a sufficient extent to allow the disease to progress, it is not of much clinical use.

Type I and Type II errors

The inequality signs $<$ and $>$ simply mean 'less than' and 'more than', so a statement that: $P < 0.05$ in relation to a hypothesis which has been tested means that if the Null Hypothesis is valid, the observed effect will arise in less than one in 20 instances. It is important to remember that the level of significance is thus the *probability of false positives,* that is, of wrongly rejecting the Null Hypothesis. This is sometimes described as an error of the first kind (Type I or α error). There is another frequent source of error, known as an error of the second kind (Type II or β error). This is the probability of accepting a Null Hypothesis when it is, in fact, invalid. This will arise particularly with small samples. Increasing the sample size reduces both Type I and Type II errors.

Incidence and prevalence
The *incidence* of a condition is the rate of occurrence of new cases. It can thus be defined as:

That fraction of the population at risk who do not initially have the condition who develop it in a given time period

or

$$\text{Incidence rate} = \frac{\text{number of new cases of a disease}}{\text{total population at risk}} \text{ per unit of time}$$

Incidence rates, apart from those for diseases like the common cold, tend to be low, and require large populations for accurate assessment.

The *prevalence* is the total number of persons with a disease or other characteristic in a defined population

or

$$\text{Prevalence} = \frac{\text{total number of existing cases}}{\text{total population}}$$

Prevalence can be expressed either as *point* prevalence, that is, at a given moment of time, or as *period* prevalence, that is, over a given period of time such as a month or a year. It therefore depends on two things:

The rate at which new cases accumulate;
The duration of the disease process

and shows the residual effect of both 'gains' (new cases) and 'losses' (deaths or recoveries). Point prevalence will thus be low for conditions which remit or can be treated rapidly, or which quickly kill.

So, for example, a particularly dangerous influenza virus could be associated with a high *incidence* of 'flu but a low point *prevalence* (because it killed off its victims quickly).

Crude and standardized rates
When we speak of birth rates or death rates, pass rates or fail rates, we

are speaking of the frequency of an observed event in relation to the total number in whom or to whom the event might occur. The choice of denominator is important. So the denominator for stillbirth rate consists of the total number of live births plus the total number of late fetal deaths at or over 28 weeks gestation, that is, the total births after 28 weeks gestation.

The *crude death rate* for any town for a particular year is the number of deaths per 1000 population, but this does not take into account the age distribution of that population. So, for example, in a town such as Eastbourne, with a high population of older, retired people, the crude death rate will be higher than that in a University town. The *standardized death rate* for age is a weighted average, which takes into account the age distribution in that town. The population is divided into arbitrary age groups, usually by 5 or 10-year intervals and the deaths per head of the population *of each age group* are calculated. The proportion of each age group in the population in Britain *as a whole* is known, so that the age-specific death rates can then be compared.

Example 1.1

In 1978 there were 5108 stillbirths out of a total of 601 526 births after 28 weeks gestation.* The crude stillbirth rate, expressed per thousand births, was thus:

$$\frac{5108}{601\ 526} \times 1000 = 8.49 \text{ per thousand births}$$

Suppose now we wish to assess the stillbirth rate standardized for the baby's sex. There were 309 722 boys and 291 804 girls born after 28 weeks that year (51.5 and 48.5% respectively). The actual numbers of stillbirths were 2634 boys and 2474 girls. The stillbirth rates per thousand thus work out at 8.50 for boys and 8.48 for girls, a minimal difference.

There are, however, some causes of stillbirth which occur more frequently in one sex than another, major congenital anomalies being a case in point. In 1978, such anomalies were recorded as the main cause of stillbirth in 381 baby boys and 669 girls. Since we know the overall numbers of stillbirths by sex, we can calculate the proportion of stillbirths related to congenital anomaly corrected for sex, which works out as:

* *Mortality statistics: childhood and maternity.* 1978. HMSO:DH3 no. 5

$$\frac{381}{2634} \times 100 = 14.5\% \text{ (boys)}$$

and

$$\frac{669}{2474} \times 100 = 27.0\% \text{ (girls)}$$

Since the total stillbirth rates were 8.50/1000 for boys and 8.48/1000 for girls, the rate per thousand for stillbirths related to congenital anomaly, standardized for sex, are:

and
$$8.50 \times 0.145 = 1.23/1000 \text{ (boys)}$$
$$8.48 \times 0.270 = 2.29/1000 \text{ (girls)}$$

2

Normal or Gaussian distribution

Basic description

Numerical data such as height and weight are examples of *continuously variable* quantities, while such numerical data as the number of living children in a family are *discontinuous* variables. When one considers a sample of either kind of data, there will be considerable individual variation within that sample. Consider, for example, the measurements in Table 2.1 of the weight in kilograms of 45 primigravidae at booking. These weights are given to the nearest kg, using the convention that rounds up from 0.5 kg, so 64.5 kg has been recorded as 65 kg; 65.4 kg would also be recorded as 65 kg.

Figure 2.1 is a *histogram* in which the area of each rectangle is directly proportional to the number of observations in each group (the *frequency*). It would also have been possible to express the frequency as the proportion of the whole sample made up by that group. So in group F, covering the range 65–69 kg, there are 7 patients out of a total of 45, or (7/45 × 100 =) 15.5%. This proportional frequency is shown on the right-hand side.

Instead of plotting the individual frequencies for each weight grouping, we could also plot a *cumulative* curve such as that in Figure

Table 2.1 Weight (kg) of 45 primigravidae at booking. The weights are grouped by 5 kg intervals, i.e. Group A ranges from 40–44 kg, Group B from 45–49 kg, and so on. The number of observations in each group is given in brackets.

A (1)	B (3)	C (6)	D (8)	E (10)	F (7)	G (4)	H (4)	I (2)
43	46	50	55	60	65	70	75	80
	46	50	56	60	66	70	76	84
	49	51	56	61	67	73	77	
		53	56	61	67	74	78	
		54	57	62	68			
		54	58	62	68			
			59	62	69			
			59	63				
				64				
				64				

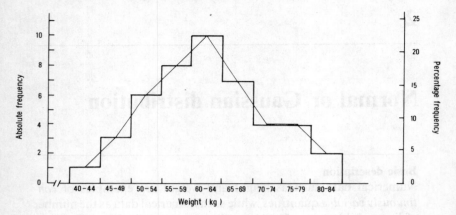

Fig. 2.1 Frequency histogram of body weight of 45 primigravidae at an antenatal booking clinic. The frequency polygon of the data is shown as (——).

2.2. Here, the point for the < 45 kg group is obviously the same as on Figure 1.1. For the next point, however, we *add* the frequency of the 45–49 kg group to that of the < 45 kg group. We are therefore saying that (1 + 3 =) 4 patients out of the 45 have weights of 49 kg or less. For the third point on the curve we add the frequency of the 50–54 kg group to that of the 45–49 and < 45 kg groups. We can now say that (1 + 3 + 6 =) 10 of the 45 patients have body weights of 54 kg or less; this is nearly a quarter of the sample. We continue to work our way

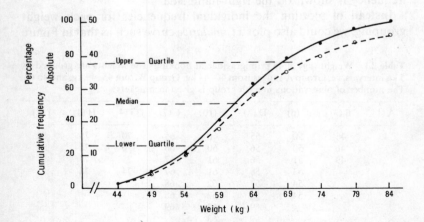

Fig. 2.2 Cumulative frequency polygon for the data of Figure 2.1. The polygon for the absolute values is shown as (- - -), that for percentage values is shown as (___).

through the sample, until all groups have been added in. This *absolute* cumulative frequency curve is shown as - - - - - on Figure 2.2.

It is of course also possible to assess each cumulative frequency as a percentage of the whole population. So for the first two weight groupings, where the absolute cumulative frequency is 4, the *percentage* cumulative frequency is $(4/45) \times 100 = 8.8\%$. The percentage cumulative frequency curve is shown as ———— on Figure 2.2.

Cumulative frequency curves are often used for such information as deaths in association with a given disease over a period of time, and allow calculation of, for example, 5-year survival rates.

The median and lower and upper *quartiles* are also shown on Figure·2.2. The *median* has the property that half the population lie below, and half above it. It is thus the 50% point. In general, it can be said that if a number (n) of measurements or observations are arranged in order of magnitude (ranked):

The median is the $(n + 1)/2$th measurement or observation.

Equation 1

Consider a very simple example:

Example 2.1
What is the median of the seven numbers 8, 5, 3, 7, 1, 2, 6?
Rank them first:

1, 2, 3, 5, 6, 7, 8

Then since $n = 7$, the median is the $(7 + 1)/2$th figure, i.e. the fourth figure, which is 5. If the number 1 were omitted, then $n = 6$ and the median would be the $(6 + 1)/2$th figure, i.e. the 3.5th figure. This is simply calculated as the mean (average) of 5 and 6 (the third and fourth figures) giving an answer of 5.5. Remember that the median itself is *not* 3.5 but the 3.5th *figure* in the ranked sample.

To return to the data of Table 2.1 and Figure 2.2, it appears that the median weight is greater than 59 and less than 64 kg. It can be calculated as being the $(45 + 1)/2 = 23$rd weight, which from Table 2.1 can be seen to be 62 kg. Similarly, the lower quartile (25% point) has the property that one quarter of the population lie below, and three quarters above it. The weight corresponding to this point will be greater than 54 and less than 59 kg and may be calculated as being the $(n + 1)/4$th figure in the ranked sample. This is the 11.5th figure, i.e. the mean of 55 and 56 kg which is 55.5 kg. Thus, we can say that a quarter of this sample weigh less than 55.5 kg.

Returning now to Figure 2.1, it can be seen that the histogram is nearly symmetrical, with the left-hand half being almost a mirror-image of the right. This is known as a *normal* or Gaussian distribution and is the basis of much descriptive and comparative statistical work. Common sense suggests that in a very large sample the irregularities as seen in Figure 2.1 would be smoothed out, as in Figure 2.3. It is possible mathematically to derive the curve which would fit the data shown in a normal curve, which is of the form:

$$y = \frac{1}{\sigma \sqrt{2\pi}} e^{-\frac{(x-\mu)^2}{2\sigma^2}}$$ Equation 2

where y is the frequency or proportion of xs in a given group, μ is the average or *mean* value overall, and σ is the *standard deviation,* a measure of scatter about the mean (see below). *Don't worry* about this intimidating equation. Basic descriptive and comparative statistics use functions derived from it which, as you will see, are perfectly straightforward. Equation 2 itself will not be used in this book.

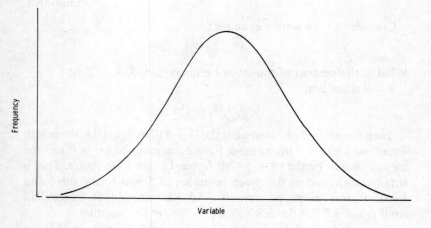

Fig. 2.3 The normal curve, as described by Equation 2. Normal distributions are bell-shaped and symmetrical about the mean value.

There is obviously a central tendency of the data in Figure 2.1, with the greatest frequency of observation occurring in group ‹E (60–64 kg). This is known as the *modal* group. Another way of expressing the central tendency is by calculating the average or mean weight. If all the individual weights in Table 2.1 were added together, and the total divided by 45, we would have a figure for the mean weight of each woman *in that sample*. This can be expressed mathematically by:

$$\bar{x} = \frac{\Sigma x}{n}$$

Equation 3

where x = any individual weight
Σ = the sum of (pronounced 'sigma')
n = the number of observations
$\bar{x}$ = the mean weight (pronounced 'x bar')

In this example, the sum of the individual measurements, Σx, is 2798 and $n = 45$ so $\bar{x} = 62.2$ kg. As Figure 2.1 shows, in a normal distribution the mean lies within the modal group.

The measurements in this example were made on a small sample of the total population of primigravidae. If we could weigh the entire population, we could measure the true population mean, known as μ (pronounced 'mew'), but almost always we have to make do with a sample.

Variance and standard deviation

A simple calculation of the sample mean, $\bar{x}$, tells us nothing about how the sample is made up. The two frequency distributions shown in Figure 2.4 would have an identical mean but the data cover differ ranges. We therefore need an estimate of the variability around the mean, which is usually expressed as the *variance*.

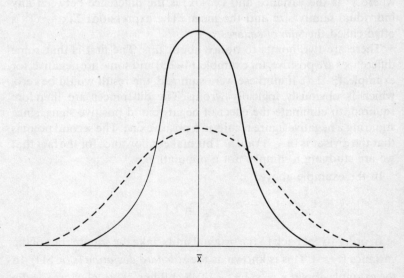

Fig. 2.4 Two normal distributions with identical mean values but different variances. The bigger variance is that of the distribution shown by broken lines (---).

Example 2.2

Consider the number of children in 6 families. In the first there are
four children, in the second there are two, in the third one, in the
fourth and fifth three, and in the sixth, two. This could also have been
shown as:

$$x_1 = 4, x_2 = 2, x_3 = 1, x_4 = 3, x_5 = 3, x_6 = 2$$

where the subscripts $_1$, $_2$, $_3$, etc., are simply arbitrary identifications of
the individual families. The mean number of children per family is
thus given by:

$$\bar{x} = \frac{4 + 2 + 1 + 3 + 3 + 2}{6} = \frac{15}{6} = 2.5 \text{ children per family}$$

The variance is then calculated as the *average* amount by which any
individual family size differs from the mean.

$$\text{variance} = \frac{(4 - 2.5)^2 + (2 - 2.5)^2 + \ldots + (2 - 2.5)^2}{n - 1}$$

This can be summarised as:

$$s^2 = \frac{\Sigma(x - \bar{x})^2}{(n - 1)} \qquad \text{Equation 4}$$

where s^2 is the variance and $(x - \bar{x})$ is the difference between any
individual family size and the mean. The expression: $\Sigma(x - \bar{x})^2$ is
often called the *sum of squares*.

There are two points to notice about this. The first is that some
differences are positive, for example, (4–2.5) and some are negative, for
example, (2–2.5). If all these were summed, the result would be zero,
which is obviously logically wrong. The differences are therefore
squared, to eliminate the effect of negative and positive signs, since
squaring a negative figure results in a positive one. The second point is
that the divisor is $(n - 1)$ *not n*. This makes allowance for the fact that
we are studying a sample, not a population.

In the example above,

$$s^2 = \frac{5.5}{5} = 1.1$$

In order to get back to the original units, take the square root of the
variance ($\sqrt{s^2}$). This is known as the *standard deviation* (*s* or SD). In
the example above, $s = \sqrt{1.1} = 1.048$ children. This, of course, is the
standard deviation about the *sample* mean, and will usually be the
measurement with which we are dealing. The standard deviation

about the true population mean is known as σ (little sigma).

It may be helpful to consider the variance and standard deviation of a sample as estimates of the *observed* differences from what would be *expected* if there were no natural variation. In Figure 2.4, it is apparent that both the variance and the standard deviation will be greater for the sample whose frequency distribution is shown as - - - - -, than for that shown as ———, although the mean values are identical.

Equation 4 can be simplified by use of the identity:

$$\Sigma(x - \bar{x})^2 = \Sigma x^2 - \frac{(\Sigma x)^2}{n}$$ Equation 5

Many simple calculators will now accumulate both Σx and Σx^2, making this calculation very straightforward. Indeed, many have a basic programme for the calculation of mean and standard deviation. Be careful about the latter measurement however. On some calculators only the function:

$$s^2 = \frac{\Sigma(x - \bar{x})^2}{n} \text{ rather than } \frac{\Sigma(x - \bar{x})^2}{(n - 1)}$$

is given. When the sample size is relatively large, (n greater than 50) the difference will be small, but where the size of a sample is itself small, the difference can become important.

Outliers
A small point here, which is worth remembering, concerns *outliers*. An isolated measurement which stands out very obviously from the rest of a sample is known as an outlier, and will, of course, have the effect in small samples of grossly distorting the mean and variance. Sometimes a clerical error is found, sometimes an error of measurement, but most often, there is no apparent explanation. If the outlier is more than $\pm 5 \times$ standard deviation away from the mean of the rest of the sample, then it is probably safe to exclude it, on the assumption that it has in fact come from another population (see below). You should however always make plain when you have done this, and be wary of doing it in small samples.

Use of tables of z (the standard normal deviate)
It can be shown both mathematically and graphically that in a normal distribution, a range of 1.96 standard deviations *on either side of the mean* will cover 95% of the area under the curve, that is, of the distribution, so that only 2.5% of the sample will lie in each 'tail'

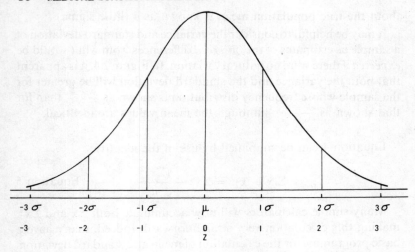

Fig. 2.5 A normal distribution of data, with a population mean of μ and a population standard deviation of σ. The area covered by the range -2σ to $+2\sigma$ is just over 95% of the total. The standard normal deviate z, is 0 at the population mean.

(Figure 2.5). Similarly, a range of 3.09 standard deviations *on either side of the mean* will cover 99.8% of the area under the curve, so that only 0.1% of the sample will lie in each 'tail'. These two important factors, 1.96 and 3.09, are frequently rounded off to 2 and 3 respectively, to allow ease of calculation. The column headed 'Special Quantiles' in Appendix 1 summarizes some frequently-used multiplication factors for defining proportions of areas under a curve of normally-distributed data in large samples ($n > 30$). This ability to determine proportionate areas under the normal curve has other uses.

Example 2.3
Imagine that you have data concerning basal heart rate in the second trimester of pregnancy from a group of 1000 women. Figure 2.6 shows that this data is normally distributed, with a mean value ($\bar{x}$) of 80 beats $\cdot$ min^{-1} and standard deviation (s) of 10. We will assume that this sample mean and standard deviation approximate to the population mean and standard deviation, μ and σ, since the sample size is large.

With this information, we can calculate the probability that any *individual's* heart rate will lie within a specified range of values. This involves assessment of the area under the normal curve covered by that particular range. Calculating areas under curves involves the use

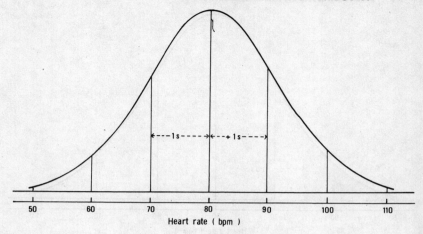

Fig. 2.6 A normal distribution of basal heart rate for women in second trimester pregnancy

of the formidable-looking Equation 2, so it is fortunate that tables such as those in Appendix 1 are available giving values for areas under a normal curve in terms of standard deviations. These are known as tables of z.

For any given value (x) of our variable, in this case heart rate, we can calculate the corresponding z-value from:

$$z = \frac{x - \bar{x}}{s}$$ Equation 6

All this is doing is calculating the *ratio* between the difference between the value of x under consideration and the mean, and the standard deviation. Tables of z then give you the area under the curve of the normal distribution represented by this ratio.

So, for example, a heart rate of 65 beats $\cdot$ min^{-1} would give a z-value of:

$$z = \frac{65 - 80}{10} = \frac{-15}{10} = -1.5$$

From Appendix 1 we can see that a z-value of -1.5 has 6.68% of the area of the curve to the left of it, i.e. 6.68% of heart rates are below this value and $(100 - 6.68 =)$ 93.32% are above it. This is illustrated as the shaded area to the left of Figure 2.7.

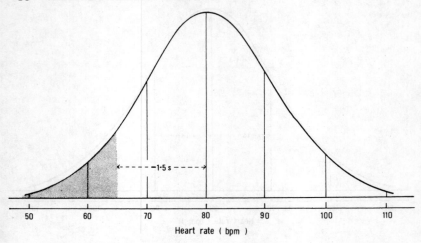

Heart rate (bpm)

Fig. 2.7 The shaded area superimposed on the normal curve of Figure 2.6 is the proportion of the total area lying at and beyond $\mu - 1.5$ standard deviations, i.e. at a z of -1.5.

Thus, to calculate the probability of an individual's heart rate lying within a specified range, say 65–85 beats $\cdot$ min^{-1}, we simply do the calculation in Equation 6 for each value and obtain the area under discussion by subtraction. We know that 6.68% of heart rates are below 65 beats $\cdot$ min^{-1}. We calculate z for 85 beats $\cdot$ min^{-1} as:

$$z = \frac{85-80}{10} = 0.5$$

A z-value of 0.5 has 69.15% of the heart rates in our sample lying below it (Appendix 1). The area for the range under discussion is therefore (69.15 − 6.68 =) 62.47%.

This means that if 100 women in second trimester pregnancy had their heart rates measured, about 62 of them would be expected to have heart rates between 65 and 85.

Cut-off points
The z-distribution is very useful in deciding cut-off points for the classification of diseases where a biochemical marker can reasonably be used.

Example 2.4
Consider, for example, the use of serum uric acid (SUA) measurements as an indicator of impending pregancy-induced hypertension (PIH), a value of 350 μmol $\cdot$ l^{-1} or more being used as a cut-off point.

This presupposes, incidentally, that concentrations of SUA are normally-distributed in both normal and hypertensive patients, which may, of course, not be true.

Imagine that in a population of normotensive women the mean SUA at 34 weeks gestation was $250 \, \mu mol \cdot l^{-1}$, with a standard deviation of 50 while in women who subsequently developed PIH, the mean value was $425 \, \mu mol \cdot l^{-1}$, with a standard deviation of 75. If we now use these figures as the basis for a predictive test, using the arbitrary cut-off point of $350 \, \mu mol \cdot l^{-1}$ we can calculate the proportion of normal women who will wrongly be classified as being at risk of developing PIH.

$$z = \frac{250 - 350}{50} = \frac{-100}{50} = -2$$

From Appendix I we can see that $\sim 2.3\%$ of normal women will be mistakenly diagnosed (*false positive*) as being at risk of developing PIH by this criterion.

Conversely,

$$z = \frac{425 - 350}{75} = \frac{75}{75} = 1$$

so 15.8% of women in the PIH group will be said *not* to be at risk. This is probably an unacceptably high proportion, so we can alter the cut-off point until we find one in which the risk of such *false-negative* values arising is acceptably low. This can be done by arbitrarily defining an acceptable false-negative rate, for example, 1%, and using Appendix I to determine the value of z which this represents. Appendix I shows that a z value of -3.10 is required in order to miss only 1% of women with PIH. Given a standard deviation of 75 for the population with PIH, this means that the cut-off point would need to be at $(425 - (3.1 \times 75) =) 192.5 \, \mu mol \cdot l^{-1}$. However, this is below the mean for the normotensive group, and a cut-off point of $192.5 \, \mu mol \cdot l^{-1}$ would thus be associated with a very high *false-positive* rate (87.5%). Logically, this tells us that SUA measurements alone are not specific enough for the adequate detection of developing PIH; they need to be combined with other measurements.

Classification

Obviously there are many factors to be considered when arriving at the diagnosis of a disease, but if considerable reliance is placed upon a cut-off point of any kind, there are various things to be remembered. In any population of patients with and without a disease, there are four possible outcomes in terms of a predictive test. A patient can be free of the disease and have a 'normal' test (possibility a); they can be free of the disease and yet have an 'abnormal' test (possibility b, a false positive test); they can have the disease but have a 'normal' test result (c, a false negative test) or they can have the disease and have an 'abnormal' test result (d). We, therefore, require a test which is both *sensitive* and *specific*.

The *sensitivity* of any test is a measure of its ability to distinguish as positive those patients who have the condition under investigation. The *specificity* is a measure of the ability correctly to identify those patients who do not have the condition. These are rather different concepts, as a *reductio ad absurdam* example will show. Suppose you took the possession of functional ovaries as a way of diagnosing pregnancy. True, you would identify correctly all pregnant women, that is, the sensitivity would be high, but since a substantial proportion of women with functional ovaries will not be pregnant, the specificity will be very low. To summarize this:

$$\text{Sensitivity} = \frac{\text{number tested as positive}}{\text{total with the condition}}$$

$$\text{Specificity} = \frac{\text{number tested as negative}}{\text{total without the condition}}$$

If we revert to the example using serum uric acid as a marker for PIH, consider a survey of 5000 pregnant women in a year.

Example 2.5

	'True' diagnosis		
SUA 350 μmol/l	Normotensive	PIH	Total
Below	4400 (a)	80 (c)	4480
Above	100 (b)	420 (d)	520
Total	4500	500	5000

$$\text{Sensitivity} = \frac{420}{500} \times 100 = 84.0\% \text{ i.e. } 16.0\% \text{ false negative}$$

This can also be expressed as:

$$\text{Sensitivity} = \frac{d}{c + d}$$

$$\text{Specificity} = \frac{4400}{4500} \times 100 = 97.7\% \text{ i.e. } 2.3\% \text{ false positive}$$

This can also be expressed as:

$$\text{Specificity} = \frac{a}{a + b}$$

Clinicians are also likely to be interested in the *predictive value* of any test classification. The predictive value of an abnormal test relates to the proportion of patients with an 'abnormal' test result who do not have the condition under investigation. The predictive value of a normal test is, of course, the converse of this, namely, the proportion of patients with a 'normal' test result who do not have the condition. Thus in Example 2.5, the predictive value of a serum uric acid measurement greater than $350 \, \mu\text{mol} \cdot \text{l}^{-1}$ is:

$$\text{Predictive value} = \frac{d}{b + d} = \frac{420}{520} \times 100 = 80.8\%$$

i.e. the predicted outcome (PIH) will occur in about four patients of every five who have serum uric acid concentrations greater than $350 \, \mu\text{mol} \cdot \text{l}^{-1}$.

The predictive value of a negative test, that is, serum uric acid concentrations less than $350 \, \mu\text{mol} \cdot \text{l}^{-1}$ is:

$$\text{Predictive value} = \frac{4400}{4480} \times 100 = 98.2\%$$

Standard errors

In medicine one usually takes a sample and extrapolates from it to describe a population. We are therefore very often interested in how representative our sample mean, $\bar{x}$, is likely to be of the true population mean, μ. When the sample is small, there is a high probability that the distribution of the members of it does not truly approximate to the distribution of the members of the population and that the sample mean differs from the population mean. If we were to take several (m) samples, under the same conditions, the average *of those sample means* would approach the true population mean, μ. This is illustrated in Figure 2.8.
Thus:

$$\mu \simeq \frac{(\bar{x}_1 + \bar{x}_2 + \bar{x}_3 + \ldots + \bar{x}_m)}{m}$$

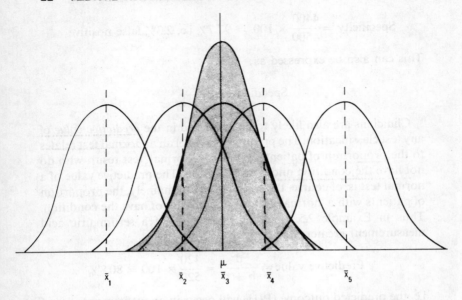

Fig. 2.8 If several samples (unshaded distributions) are taken from a normally-distributed population, the mean value of the sample means ($\bar{x}_1, ..., \bar{x}_5$ in this example) will give a more representative idea of the population mean (shaded distribution).

Note that we are now averaging the *means* of our *m* samples which will cluster around the true population mean.

Example 2.6
Suppose that you have taken 6 samples each of 5 measurements of blood glucose concentration (mmol $\cdot$ l^{-1}), summarized below:

		$\bar{x}$	s^2	s
Sample 1	4,5,6,6,5	5.2	0.7	0.836
Sample 2	3,7,4,4,6	4.8	2.7	1.643
Sample 3	5,4,3,6,4	4.4	1.3	1.140
Sample 4	5,4,5,4,6	4.8	0.7	0.836
Sample 5	6,4,5,5,5	5.0	0.5	0.707
Sample 6	5,4,3,5,6	4.6	1.3	1.140

The means of the samples can themselves be seen to be clustering around the overall mean, which is 4.80 mmol $\cdot$ l^{-1}. If we now calculate the average of these sample means, we find:

$$\bar{x}_m = \frac{(5.2 + 4.8 + 4.4 + 4.8 + 5.0 + 4.6)}{6} = 4.80$$

with variance 0.080, which is substantially smaller than any of the individual variances. The sample means are themselves normally distributed around the true population mean, and have a deviation from it which can be calculated as:

$$s_m = \sqrt{\frac{s_m^2}{m}} \text{ or } \frac{s_m}{\sqrt{m}} \text{ (the same thing)} \qquad \text{Equation 7}$$

To avoid confusion, this deviation from the estimated population (rather than sample) mean, is usually described as the *standard error* of the mean.

It is however frequently not possible or practicable to get several samples from a population and we want to assess how closely our sample mean approaches the population mean. To do this, we substitute our known sample variance, s^2, for the unknown population variance, s_m^2. Thus:

$$SE = \sqrt{\frac{s^2}{n}} \text{ or } \frac{s}{\sqrt{n}} \qquad \text{Equation 8}$$

and, of course, depends on sample size.

Example 2.7
Suppose that you have measured serum potassium concentrations in 4 children with Bartter's syndrome, and found the mean value to be $1.8 \text{ mmol} \cdot \text{l}^{-1}$, with a standard deviation of $1 \text{ mmol} \cdot \text{l}^{-1}$. The standard error is then calculated as:

$$SE = \frac{1}{\sqrt{4}} = 0.5$$

If you now accumulate data from a further 21 children with Bartter's syndrome, n is increased to 25. Assume s stays at 1, then:

$$SE = \frac{1}{\sqrt{25}} = 0.2$$

If you now increase your sample size to 100 and s stays at 3:

$$SE = \frac{1}{\sqrt{100}} = 0.1$$

Thus, when n is small, the standard error will be relatively large. The effect of n rapidly diminishes in large samples, which are that much more likely to be representative of the population as a whole.

Increasing the sample size to 900 in the example above would only alter the standard error to 0.03.

Confidence intervals

Earlier in this chapter, we saw that in a normal distribution, a range of ± 1.96 standard deviations on either side of the mean will cover 95% of the area under the curve. In large samples, in which $n > 30$, we can calculate what are called 95% confidence limits using the mean and its associated standard error. This gives us information about the range of values within which the true population mean is likely to lie.

The 95% confidence limits are given as the mean value ± 1.96 times the standard error. This means that there is a 95% chance that the true population mean will lie within the calculated range. Appendix I is used again to give the appropriate factors by which the SE must be multiplied for other, frequently-used, confidence limits.

Example 2.8

The standard deviation of the weights in Table 2.1 can be calculated as 9.7 kg with a mean of 62.2 kg. Since $n = 45$, the standard error is:

$$SE = \frac{9.7}{\sqrt{45}} = 1.45$$

The 95% confidence interval is therefore $62.2 \pm (1.96 \times 1.45)$ or 59.3–65.0 kg. There is only 1 chance in 20 that the true population mean lies outside this range.

Coefficient of variation

One last concept before we leave the basics of the normal distribution is the concept of the *coefficient of variation*. This, which is also known as the coefficient of error, is given by:

$$COV = \frac{s}{\bar{x}} \times 100\% \qquad \text{Equation 9}$$

This simply expresses the standard deviation as a proportion of the mean. Obviously the coefficient of variation of the distribution shown as ----- in Figure 2.4 will be bigger than that of the distribution shown as ———.

The coefficient of variation is useful in the comparison of assay results from different laboratories, and as a measure of the confidence which one can place in any individual assay. For example, if serum ACTH was measured in an identical reference sample 12 times in laboratory A and 12 times in laboratory B, and laboratory A sent back a mean result of $17.5 \, ng \cdot l^{-1}$, s $2.5 \, ng \cdot l^{-1}$ while laboratory B sent back a mean result of $19.0 \, ng \cdot l^{-1}$, s $5.0 \, ng \cdot l^{-1}$, the two coefficients of variation would be 14.2% and 26.3% respectively. If there were no other factors to be considered, one would 'trust' any results for ACTH measurement from laboratory A more than those from laboratory B. It is obvious that this is the same kind of information as that given by confidence limits, but expressed in a different way.

Skewed distribution

The normal curve shown in Figure 2.1 is fairly easy to handle, but in practice, biological data often has a skewed distribution.

Example 2.9
55 women presented at an antenatal clinic. 7 were nulliparous, 23 were primips, 14 had two children, 4 had three children, 2 had four children, 2 had five children, 1 had 6 children, 1 had seven and 1 had eight children. Figure 2.9 shows the distribution curve for this sample. It will be seen that instead of the symmetry of Figure 2.1, there is now a long 'tail' to the right of the modal class, which is, of course, the primiparous group. In this example, the mean number of children is given by:

$$\bar{x} = \frac{[(7 \times 0) + (23 \times 1) + (14 \times 2) + \ldots + (1 \times 8)]}{55}$$

= 1.85 children/woman with a standard deviation of 1.70.

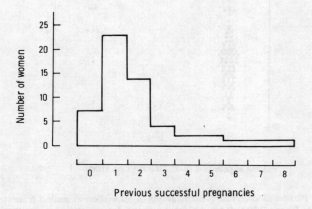

Fig. 2.9 Frequency histogram of the number of previous successful pregnancies in 55 women presenting at an antenatal clinic

This mean has been 'pulled up' by the long tail. The 95% confidence limits range from 1.4 to 2.3 children, which is not very helpful information. Under these circumstances, it is *inappropriate* to calculate the mean and variance, and the appropriate descriptive statistics are the modal class and the median. In this example, the modal class is the second, primiparity. The median number of children will be the $(55 + 1)/2$th number, that is the 28th. We know

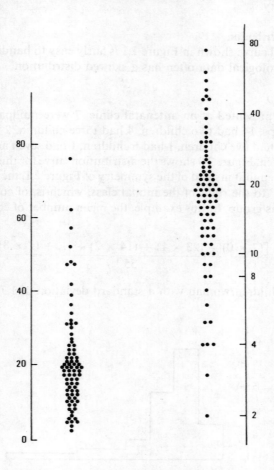

Plasma aldosterone concentration (ng. 100ml^{-1})

Fig. 2.10 Plasma aldosterone concentrations in 80 women in second trimester pregnancy. Figure 2.10 (left hand side) shows the data plotted on an arithmetic scale Figure 2.10 (right hand side) shows the same data plotted on a logarithmic$_{10}$ scale.

that there are 7 nulliparae and 23 primiparae. The 28th number will therefore be in the primiparous group.

There is another way of dealing with skewed data, which is to *transform* it. Probably the most commonly-used transformation for biological data is to convert the data to $\log_{10}$ values. Semilogarithmic graph paper, which has one linear ('ordinary') axis, and one on $\log_{10}$ is readily available. This allows you to plot out your basic data without using $\log_{10}$ tables, and thus lets you see at a glance whether conversion to $\log_{10}$ will in fact normalise the distribution of your data. Figure 2.10 illustrates the use of such paper for data concerning plasma aldosterone measurements in 80 women in second trimester pregnancy. The left hand side of Figure 2.10 shows that the data is skewed, but it is evident from the right hand side of the Figure that the use of $\log_{10}$ values will substantially normalise the distribution of this data. A method of confirming this visual impression is given in Chapter 3, in the section 'Use of χ^2 to determine goodness of fit'.

SUMMARY OF CHAPTER 2

1. When data are normally distributed, the left hand side of the frequency distribution is an approximate mirror image of the right hand side.
2. Under these circumstances, the mean ($\bar{x}$; Equation 3) and median (Equation 1) lie within the modal group.
3. The median of a sample has half of the sample lying below, and half above it. The lower quartile has the lowest quarter of the data lying below it, while the upper quartile has the highest quarter lying above it.
4. The variance (s^2; Equation 4) and standard deviation (s) of a sample are measures of the scatter of data around the sample mean. The smaller they are, the less natural variation is present in the sample.
5. 95% of the area under a normal distribution curve lies within the range of the mean plus or minus 1.96 times the standard deviation. 99% lies within the range of the mean ± 2.58 times the standard deviation.
6. If an outlier (a single, isolated measurement) is more than ± 5 times the standard deviation away from the sample mean, it is reasonable to conclude that it is from a different population, and exclude it from further calculations.
7. Tables of z, (the standard normal deviate) can be used to calculate the probability of any individual value lying within a specified range of data (Equation 6) and to decide cut-off points for the

classification of disease. Other uses are mentioned in subsequent chapters.

8. The sensitivity of any test for a disease is a measure of its ability to distinguish as 'positive' those patients who have the condition. The specificity is a measure of the ability correctly to identify those patients who do not have the condition.

9. The standard error (SE; Equation 8) of a sample is dependent upon the sample size and is used as an index of how closely the sample mean approximates to the population mean. ✳

10. Confidence intervals are used to give the probability of the true ✳ population mean lying within a range derived from a sample mean and its standard error. Thus there is a 5% chance of the true population mean lying outside the range: $\bar{x} \pm (1.96 \times SE)$ and a 1% chance of it lying outside the range: $\bar{x} \pm (2.58 \times SE)$.

11. The coefficient of variation (Equation 9) expresses the standard deviation as a percentage of the mean. It is widely used in the assessment of laboratory results.

12. When the left- and right-hand sides of a frequency distribution do not approximate to mirror images, the data is said to be skewed. It is inappropriate to calculate the mean and standard deviation of such data. The median value and the mode are then the appropriate indices of central tendency.

13. It is frequently possible to transform skewed data by expressing it as $\log_{10}$ or $\ln$; other transformations are also possible. Once the data is normalised, its mean and standard deviation can be calculated as usual.

QUESTIONS FOR CHAPTER 2

Q1. A GP found from his records that, of 100 female patients between 25–40 years old presenting consecutively at his surgery, 19 came once in the year, 29 came twice, 22 came three times, 18 came four times and the remainder came five times. What is the mean number of visits per year by these patients?

A1. The mean ($\bar{x}$) is given by Equation 3. Σx can be calculated by multiplying the number of patients in any group by the number of times they came.

Thus $\Sigma x = (19 \times 1) + (29 \times 2) + (22 \times 3) + (18 \times 4) + (12 \times 5)$

$= 275$

We know $n = 100$, so

$\bar{x} = 275/100 = 2.75$ visits per year

Q2. The mean fasting blood glucose concentration in 49 normal males was found to be 4.0 mmol $\cdot$ l^{-1}, variance 0.09 mmol $\cdot$ l^{-1}, 95% of this sample will lie within one of these ranges; which one?

(a) 3.4–4.6 mmol $\cdot$ l^{-1}
(b) 2–6 mmol $\cdot$ l^{-1}
(c) 3.1–4.9 mmol $\cdot$ l^{-1}

A2. Range (a) which has been calculated from $\bar{x} \pm 2s$, remembering that s, the standard deviation, is the square root of the variance. In this example, we are concerned with the sample itself, and not with the total population. - s = standard deviation

Q3. 250 medical students sat an examination marked out of 100. The mean mark obtained was 61, standard deviation 10. Since the pass mark was 50, how many students failed?

A3.

$$z = \frac{50 - 61}{10} = \frac{-11}{10} = -1.1 \qquad \text{Equation 6}$$

From Appendix I we find that 13.57% of students will have gained marks of less than 50. Since 250 students sat the exam, 34 will have failed.

Q4. It was felt to be appropriate to pass 75% of candidates in a final professional examination. From previous years the average mark obtained in this examination was known to be 68%, with a standard deviation of 14. What must the pass mark be set at?

A4. If 75% of candidates pass, 25% will fail. Appendix I shows that z must be -0.674 for this to happen.

$$\frac{? - 68}{14} = -0.674$$

$$? = 68 + (14 \times -0.674) = 58.6\%$$

The pass mark should therefore be set at 59%.

Q5. The mean serum creatinine concentration in a group of 64 normal patients was found to be $76\,\mu\text{mol} \cdot \text{l}^{-1}$, variance $25\,\mu\text{mol} \cdot \text{l}^{-1}$. What is the standard error of this mean value?

A5. Standard error is given by

$$\text{SE} = \frac{s}{\sqrt{n}} \quad \text{or} \quad \sqrt{\frac{s^2}{n}} \qquad \qquad \text{Equation 8}$$

$$= \frac{5}{8} \quad \text{or} \quad \sqrt{\frac{25}{64}} = 0.625\,\mu\text{mol} \cdot \text{l}^{-1}$$

Q6. Using the data of Q2, calculate the range within which the true population mean will fall in 98% of similar samples.

A6. From Appendix I, we see that 98% of the area under the normal curve is covered by the range $\bar{x} \pm (2.33 \times s)$. In this question we are interested in the population mean, so the estimate of s that we use is the standard error.
Thus:

$$\text{SE} = \sqrt{\frac{0.09}{49}} = 0.04$$

The 98% confidence limits are thus:

$$4.0 \pm (2.33 \times 0.04) = 3.91 - 4.09\,\text{mmol} \cdot \text{l}^{-1}$$

Q7. The lecithin/sphingomyelin (L/S) ratio was determined in amniotic fluid samples taken not more than 3 days prior to delivery from a group of 430 high risk pregnant women. An L/S ratio greater than 2 was used as an index of fetal lung maturity. Following delivery, 356 infants had no respiratory problems, although an L/S ratio of less than 2 had been recorded in 29 of them. Seventy-four infants developed respiratory problems, of whom 69% had had L/S ratios below 2. What are the sensitivity and predictive value of this test for the development of respiratory problems?

A7. The easiest way of working through this is to construct a table of the kind shown in Example 2.5. Remember that you need to calculate 69% of 74 to arrive at the number of infants with L/S ratios < 2 who developed respiratory problems.

Diagnosis L/S ratio	No respiratory problems	Respiratory problems	
> 2	327	23	350
≤ 2	29	51	80
	356	74	430

The sensitivity is then given by:

$$\text{sensitivity} = \frac{51}{51 + 23} \times 100 = 68.9\%$$

(proportion of those to resp dis.)

The predictive value for the development of respiratory problems is given by:

$$\text{predictive value} = \frac{51}{51 + 29} \times 100 = 63.7\%$$

(proportion of those with abnormal tests)

3

Other distributions

The binomial distribution

The binomial distribution is another frequently encountered distribution of data. This will occur whenever the possession or lack of a particular attribute in a population is what is being investigated. For example, any question which can be answered either 'Yes' or 'No' will give rise to a binomial distribution of data, as will, say, 'Cured' or 'Died', 'Male' or 'Female'. This distribution has the special property that if the proportion (p) of a sample falling in one category is known, then the proportion in the other category can be directly calculated, since this will be $(1 - p)$. For example, if 25 out of a random sample of 100 adults (a proportion of a quarter or 0.25) are smokers, $(1 - 0.25 =)$ 0.75 or 75% *must* be non-smokers.

Example 3.1

A random sample of 100 men were asked whether they were smokers; 43 said that they were. From this we *infer* that 43% of the total male population were smokers *at that time*. This is a *point estimate*, suggesting that *on average* there will be 43 smokers in every 100 men sampled. However, if we take several samples each of 100 men, we would not rationally expect all of them to contain 43 smokers. Common sense tells us that if we average out the numbers of men who smoke in our various samples, this average or mean value is likely to be a better representation of the true proportion (known as π) of smokers *in the population*. We may wish to know how closely the original count of 43 in 100 is likely to approach this true proportion. An equation of the form:

$$\text{standard deviation of } p \ (s_p) = \sqrt{\frac{p \times (1 - p)}{n}} \qquad \text{Equation 10}$$

where n is the number in the sample, can be used for this. The similarities between Equations 8 and 10 are obvious. The concept of a 'standard deviation of (from) the true population mean' (the standard error) has been discussed in the section on the normal distribution in Chapter 2, in which it was shown to be an estimate of how closely the mean of data from any sample is likely to approach the true population mean.

In the example described above, $p = 43/100 = 0.43$, and $(1 - p) = (1 - 0.43) = 0.57$, while $n = 100$. The standard deviation from the true population mean is then:

$$s_p = \sqrt{\frac{0.43 \times 0.57}{100}} = 0.050$$

The 95% confidence interval can then be calculated by multiplying s_p by 1.96, giving a value of 0.098. This is then both added to, and subtracted from, our original estimate of 0.43, giving a range of 0.332–0.528. Translating this back from proportions to actual figures, gives us a range of 33.2–52.8 men. Since fractional men are an absurdity, rounding off, we can quote 95% confidence intervals of 33–53 men. This means that if we were to take repeated samples of 100 men, in 95% of them between 33 and 53 men would be smokers.

The similarities between Equations 8 and 10 result from the fact that when n is greater than 30, the binomial distribution can be shown to approximate to the normal distribution. A practical point should be borne in mind, however. In Example 3.1, in which n was 100 and p was 0.43, s_p was small in relation to p (0.05 compared with 0.43, 11.6%). If our sample had consisted of 100 men who had suffered myocardial infarcts, and who had been counselled to stop smoking, we might have arrived at a point estimate of only 4 smokers in this sample ($p = 0.04$). The s_p would then be 0.019, which is much higher in relation to p (48.9%) indicating that we should place much less reliance on the point estimate as a reflection of the true smoking habits of this population. To get back to a coefficient of error of 11.6%, we would need a sample size of 1800. This is a mathematical example of the logical concept that, when p is small, large sample sizes are required to be able to assess the true population incidence. Minimal sample sizes ($n > 30$) are acceptable when p approaches 0.5, but a sample size of at least 100 is needed before the same degree of confidence can be attached to estimates of $p = 0.2$.

Example 3.2

Suppose that a medical student making a differential white cell count finds that 70 out of 250 white cells are lymphocytes. He wants to know how wide the 95% confidence interval is for such data. He first calculates the proportion of lymphocytes in the sample ($70/250 =$)

0.28 or 28%. The non-lymphocyte proportion is thus $(1 - 0.28 =)$ 0.72. The s_p is calculated as:

$$s_p = \sqrt{\frac{0.28 \times 0.72}{250}} = 0.028$$

The 95% confidence interval is thus:

$$0.28 \pm 0.055 = 0.225 - 0.335$$

This is statistical shorthand for the statement:

'In 95% of differential white cell counts, in which 250 white cells at a time are examined, the proportion of lymphocytes will range between 23 and 34%.'

Note that in this example, s_p was small in relation to p, since it was 0.028 compared with 0.28, a coefficient of variation of 10%. If only 50 white cells had been counted, of which 14 were lymphocytes, the *proportion* of lymphocytes $(14/50 =) 0.28$ would have been the same, but s_p would have been much bigger

$$s_p = \sqrt{\frac{0.28 \times 0.72}{50}} = 0.063$$

giving a coefficient of variation of 22.5%, with a 95% confidence interval of:

$$0.28 \pm 0.123 = 0.157 - 0.403$$

This is, of course, a much wider range and again illustrates the importance of sample size.

This kind of estimation can be of practical use. Suppose, having done numerous similar white cell counts giving very similar results, the student now did a differential white cell count on another sample of 250 white cells and found only 50 lymphocytes, a mere $(50/250 =)$ 20%. He knows that *from his data* he would expect to see between 23 and 34% lymphocytes in 95% of samples. This latest sample thus lies outside the 95% confidence interval, and is therefore said to be *statistically* significantly different from the general population under study at the 5% level. Of course, on an average of 5 times in 100, or 1 in 20, this assumption will be wrong, because 5% of the general population lie outside the range covered by the mean ± 1.96 standard deviations (Type I error).

As the student examined the latter sample, he was, whether consciously or unconsciously, proposing the Null Hypothesis:

'This sample comes from the same population as the other samples which I have examined' or, more formally:

'The Null Hypothesis states that the observed frequency of lymphocytes in the white cell count will not differ significantly from the expected frequency.'

The results from the last sample fell outside the 95% confidence interval, so that the Null Hypothesis was rejected, and the _Alternative Hypothesis_ (H_1), that the sample came from a different population, was accepted.

There are some instances in which actual proportions in a population are known. The total number of children vaccinated for whooping coughs in any year is known in relation to the total number of children. We can thus put an actual figure on π, the true proportion of children being vaccinated. If numerous samples each of 500 children are obtained, then the proportions of children found to be being vaccinated in these samples will cluster round the true population proportion with a standard deviation, σ_p (little sigma p) given by:

$$\sigma_p = \sqrt{\frac{\pi \times (1 - \pi)}{500}}$$

Note that this is identical in format to Equation 10, but relates specifically to the true proportion, π, in the population.

Example 3.3

The primary failure rate of recompression in air for the treatment of severe decompression sickness was known to be 47% in 1964. When recompression in oxygen was introduced, there were only 2 primary failures in the first 50 patients studied. Was treatment in oxygen exerting a significantly different effect?

H_0: Recompression in oxygen was not associated with an alteration in response.

If H_0 is valid, the failure rate following treatment in oxygen should lie within ± 1.96 standard deviations of the overall proportion, 0.47 or 47%.

$$\sigma_p = \sqrt{\frac{0.47 \times (1 - 0.47)}{50}} = 0.070$$

The 95% confidence limits are thus:

$$0.47 \pm 0.137 = 0.333 - 0.607$$

The observed failure rate after recompression in oxygen was actually 4% or 0.04, which was very substantially outside the 95% confidence limits. We can therefore confidently reject H_0.

Another development of a binomial distribution is that given by a simple recessive gene.

Example 3.4

A husband and wife are both heterozygous for albinism. This can be expressed as:

$$♂ Aa \qquad ♀ Aa$$

By simple Mendelian genetics, it can be seen that the possible genotypes for the children of such a marriage are AA, Aa, Aa, aa. Thus *on average,* 1 child in 4 will be born an albino, provided that albinism is not associated with some deleterious intrauterine effect. (This of course is an example of the care which has to be exercised when drawing conclusions from statistics.) Suppose that the parents sought advice on the likelihood of one child being born albino if they were to have 2 children. The chance of any *individual* child being homozygous (aa) is 1 in 4. There are thus 3 out of 4 chances of it being *phenotypically* normal. The second child will not be affected by the genotype of the first. There are therefore $(3/4 \times 3/4 =) 9/16$ chances of both being phenotypically normal, and $(1/4 \times 1/4 =) 1/16$ chances of both being albino. The remaining probability, 6/16, is that one will be normal and one albino.

The overall underlying theory for binomial distributions can thus be summarised as:

Individuals in a sample may possess a certain character with a probability p, or may fail to possess it with a probability $(1 - p)$. In the example above, $p = 1/4$ or 0.25. This can be expanded for use with *multinomial* and *poisson distributions*. These are considerably more specialized and will not be considered here.

The chi-squared (χ^2) distribution

Example 3.5

Carrying on from the example above, imagine that you found 100 families with both parents Aa heterozygotes, each with 2 children. In 54 families both were normal, in 8 both were albino and in 38 one child was normal and one albino. From this we can construct a table of 'observed' and 'expected' values.

The 'expected' number can be calculated from the binomial distribution given above. Thus *on average* $(9/16 \times 100) = 56.25$ families would be *expected* to have two phenotypically normal

| | Number of affected children | | | Total |
	0	1	2	
Observed number of families	54	38	8	100
Expected number of families	56.25	37.5	6.25	100

children and $(1/16 \times 100) = 6.25$ families to have two albino children.

In this example, common sense says that the observed and expected values are very close. This is not however always the case, and we might wish to put a numerical value on how closely or otherwise, the observed and expected values agree. We might wish to do this to test, for example, whether homozygosity for albinism was associated with physiological disadvantage, evidenced by there being fewer albinos observed in a population (sample) than would be expected. The hypothesis takes the form:

H_0: The proportion of albinos in the population is in accordance with that predicted by Mendelian theory

To test this hypothesis, we need to know both by how much the observations differ from the expected population means and also whether this difference is more than might reasonably be expected to occur in sampling. To assess this, a χ^2 (*chi-squared*, pronounced 'ki-squared') test is used.

First, calculate by how much the observed frequencies (O) differ from the expected (E). This can be expressed as ($O - E$). Because some of the differences will be negative, this difference is then squared, thus removing the negative sign. Each difference is then divided by the expected number, to allow for group size, thus giving an 'average difference per unit group'. These 'averages' are then added together. The resultant figure is known as χ^2. This can be expressed as:

$$\chi^2 = \sum \frac{(O - E)^2}{E} \qquad \text{Equation 11}$$

Obviously, the smaller the difference between the observed and the expected values, the smaller will χ^2 be. In the example above,

$$\chi^2 = \frac{(54 - 56.25)^2}{56.25} + \frac{(38 - 37.5)^2}{37.5} + \frac{(8 - 6.25)^2}{6.25} = 0.5866$$

Tables of χ^2 are available (Appendix 2) which show the probability of the calculated χ^2 having arisen from a sample conforming to the hypothetical model. To use this table, it is necessary to know the *number of degrees of freedom* available. In an instance such as the example quoted above, this is very easy. There are three possible *groups,* AA, Aa and aa, whose predicted frequency of occurrence has been calculated. In any sample containing a mixture of these three genotypes, once the number of AA and the number of Aa individuals is known, the number of aa individuals is fixed. So in the example above, in the sample of 100 families, once it was found that 54 had no affected children and 8 had two affected children, the number of families with 1 affected child had to be $(100 - 54 - 8 =)$ 38. There are thus 2 degrees of freedom in this example.

In other words:

If a sample of known size is classified into g groups, then there are $(g - 1)$ degrees of freedom.

Appendix 2 shows that, for 2 degrees of freedom, χ^2 would have to be *at least* 5.99 for the result to suggest that the departure from predicted values was so large as to be statistically significant, at the five per cent level. Our calculated χ^2 of 0.5866 is much smaller than this, so that we can confidently say that the observed distribution conforms well with that expected by Mendelian theory. The Null Hypothesis has therefore been accepted.

The χ^2 test of *goodness of fit* to any predicted pattern is only one example of a χ^2 test. Others will be discussed later. It is however important to remember that:

(i) The *expected* number in any group should not be less than 5.
     If it is, two groups can frequently be pooled.
(ii) The *total* number of observations should not be less than 20.
(iii) χ^2 tests *must* be carried out on actual numbers, *not* percentages.

This last point can perhaps most easily be understood with an example.

Example 3.6
A GP carried out a survey of the incidence of the common cold in his practice. Of 800 patients presenting consecutively with colds, 440 were men and 360 were women. Do these results support a hypothesis that more men get colds than women?

H_0: There is no gender-related difference in the incidence of the common cold

If H_0 is valid, the doctor would expect half his patients to be men and half women. In a sample of 800, this means that $f_{ex} = 400$ for each sex. χ^2 is thus given by:

$$\chi^2 = \frac{(+40^2)}{400} + \frac{(-40)^2}{400} = 4 + 4 = 8$$

Here we have only one degree of freedom, since, given that we know the total sample size, once we know the number of men in the sample, the number of women is determined. Appendix 2 then shows that with one degree of freedom, the probability of getting a χ^2 bigger than 8 by chance is between 1 in 100 and 1 in 1000. We therefore reject the Null Hypothesis, and arrive at an Alternative Hypothesis, namely that:

'There is a gender-related difference in the incidence of the common cold.'

Now imagine that the GP had only sampled 80 patients presenting consecutively with a cold, of whom 44 were men and 36 were women. Note that the *proportions* of men and women in the sample are identical.

$$\chi^2 = \frac{(+4)^2}{40} + \frac{(-4)^2}{40} = 0.4 + 0.4 = 0.8$$

As Appendix 2 shows, a χ^2 of this value will be arrived at by chance more than 1 in 5 times. We would therefore accept the original Null Hypothesis, from this data.

If we had only been told that '55% were men and 45% were women', *without being told the sample size*, we could not have carried out the χ^2 test, since we would have had no idea of the denominator.

In passing, this example shows again how cautious one must be in assigning biological significance to statistical data. Perhaps most of the women with colds had young families and did not want to go to surgery. Perhaps a virulent virus had chosen just that period to go through a factory where the majority of men worked. Perhaps, even, men were more concerned about their colds than women. It would need much more than one such sample to be sure that men were more susceptible to colds than women, regardless of how high the statistical significance was.

χ^2 and goodness-of-fit
In Example 3.5, a χ^2 test was used to examine whether the observed distribution of albino children fitted with that expected from the binomial distribution. This can also be done to test whether data follow a normal distribution. We know that, by using tables of z

(Appendix 1) we can predict the area under a normal curve falling on either side of any given measurement from the sample making up that curve (refer back to Figure 2.5 if you don't remember this). From this we can calculate the number of observations which we would *expect* to occur within any range of values *if the distribution were normal*. The χ^2 test then lets us test whether the observed frequencies differ significantly from the expected.

Example 3.7
Consider again the data on aldosterone concentrations in Figure 2.10. We have said, on the basis of visual inspection, that is a skewed distribution. Visual inspection is usually adequate, but working through the χ^2 test for this example allows us both formally to demonstrate that the data is not normally-distributed as it stands, and that the $\log_{10}$ transformation normalises it.

In order to draw out the frequency histogram, the data have already been grouped as: 0–9, 10–19, 20–29, etc., $ng \cdot dl^{-1}$. These are shown in Table 3.1. The arithmetic mean for this data is 21.1 ng aldosterone $\cdot dl^{-1}$, standard deviation 13.93. If the data were normally distributed, we should expect the 0–9 ng aldosterone $\cdot dl^{-1}$ group to have 19.77% of the observations falling in it. This is calculated using Equation 6.

$$z = \frac{9 - 21.1}{13.93} = -0.86$$

Appendix 1 shows that the area to the left of -0.86 is 0.1977 (19.77%). We therefore expect 19.77% of our sample of 80 (15.81) values to lie within this group. Similarly, for the group 10–19 ng aldosterone $\cdot dl^{-1}$

$$z = \frac{19 - 21.1}{13.93} = -0.15$$

The *total* area to the left of this is 44.04%, but we know that 19.77% lies within the 0–9 ng $\cdot dl^{-1}$ group. The 10–19 ng $\cdot dl^{-1}$ group thus covers $(44.04 - 19.77 =)$ 24.27%, which is equivalent to 19.41 actual measurements. This procedure is worked through for each group, as shown in Table 3.1. Note that the groups > 40 ng $\cdot dl^{-1}$ have been collapsed, to ensure that the lowest expected frequency is not less than 5. Ideally also, one should have 12 or more groups, but this is obviously limited by sample size.

The total, 12.62, of the column headed $\frac{\text{'}(O - E)^2\text{'}}{E}$ is, of course, χ^2.

Table 3.1 χ^2 test of goodness of fit for the untransformed data of Figure 2.10

Plasma aldosterone $(ng \cdot dl^{-1})$	Observed frequency	Expected frequency	$\dfrac{(O-E)^2}{E}$
0–9	13	15.81	0.499
10–19	32	19.41	8.166
20–29	19	21.47	0.284
30–39	8	15.55	3.665
> 40	8	7.76	0.007
Totals	80	80	12.621

We have calculated two parameters, $\bar{x}$ and s, to arrive at our expected values. Under these circumstances, the number of degrees of freedom is given by:

$$df = 5 \text{ (groups)} - 1 - 2 \text{ (parameters)} = 2$$

Appendix 2 shows that for two degrees of freedom, a χ^2 of 12.622 is statistically significant, $p < 0.01$. We thus reject the Null Hypothesis:

H_0: The data concerning plasma aldosterone concentrations fit a normal distribution curve

and consider that they fit some other, unspecified, distribution.

If we now apply the same test to the transformed data, as shown in Table 3.2, we arrive at a value of χ^2 of 0.526, which is not significant. We can therefore accept the null hypothesis:

H_0: The distribution of data concerning plasma aldosterone concentrations expressed as $\log_{10}$ does not differ from a normal distribution curve.

Table 3.2 χ^2 test of goodness of fit for the data of Figure 2.10 as $\log_{10}$, with $\bar{x} = 1.23$ and $s = 0.2996$ ng $\cdot$ dl^{-1}

$\log_{10}$ plasma aldosterone $(ng \cdot dl^{-1})$	Observed frequency	Expected frequency	$\dfrac{(O-E)^2}{E}$
< 0.95	13	13.68	0.033
0.96–1.27	32	31.08	0.027
1.28–1.46	19	17.10	0.211
1.47–1.59	8	8.92	0.094
> 1.60	8	9.22	0.161
Totals	80	80	0.526

SUMMARY OF CHAPTER 3

1. A binomial distribution occurs whenever the possession or lack of a particular attribute is under investigation. Individuals in a sample possess the attribute with a probability p, or fail to possess it with a probability $1 - p$.

2. Confidence intervals can be assessed as for the normal distribution when n, the number in the sample, is more than 30 and p approximates to 0.5. Sample size should be increased as p diminishes, to approximately 100 for $p = 0.2 > 0.8$. The standard deviation of p, s_p, is given by Equation 10.

3. The χ^2 statistic (Equation 11; Appendix 2) can be used to assess whether an observed binomial or other distribution accords with that expected either on the basis of knowledge of true population parameters, or on theoretical grounds.

4. When χ^2 has been calculated for g groups, there are $(g - 1)$ degrees of freedom.

5. When calculating χ^2, the expected number in any group should not be less than 5, the total number of observations should not be less than 20 and actual numbers, *not* ratios or percentages, must be used.

QUESTIONS FOR CHAPTER 3

Q1. 250 women with fluctuating symptomatology were treated with a prostaglandin synthetase inhibitor for premenstrual syndrome. 58% reported an improvement in symptoms. Is this a statistically-significant result?

A1. H_0: Treatment is not having any effect on the premenstrual symptoms

From H_0, 125 women would be expected to report an improvement in symptoms. In fact 145 did so (58% of 250). There is thus an excess of 20 women who are feeling better, and a deficit of 20 women feeling worse.

$$\chi^2 = \frac{(+20)^2}{125} + \frac{(-20)^2}{125} = 3.2 + 3.2 = 6.4$$

From Appendix 2, a χ^2 of 6.4 with 1 degree of freedom will occur less than one in 20 times on the Null Hypothesis. We therefore reject H_0, and consider that the treatment is having a statistically-significant effect.

Q2. 1050 of the 5108 reported stillbirths in 1978 were associated with congenital anomalies. A paediatric pathologist who studied 400 consecutive stillbirths in his area, found 94 of them to be associated with congenital anomaly. Does this data suggest an increased rate of congenital anomaly in his area?

A2. H_0: The congenital anomaly rate is the same in the sample as in the general population

The population proportion, π, with congenital anomaly is $(1050/5108 =) 0.205$. $(1 - \pi)$ is thus $(1 - 0.205 =) 0.795$.

$$\sigma_p = \sqrt{\frac{0.205 \times 0.795}{400}} = 0.020$$

The 95% confidence interval is:

$$0.205 \pm 0.0392 = 0.165 - 0.244$$

The anomaly rate in the sample is $(94/400 =) 0.235$. This thus lies within the 95% confidence interval, implying that the sample has almost certainly come from the normal population. We can accept the Null Hypothesis.

Q3. In Example 1.1, the stillbirth rate in association with congenital anomaly, corrected for gender, was 1.23 per thousand for boys and 2.29 per thousand for girls. Given that there were a total of 309 722 boys and 291 804 girls born that year, calculate χ^2 for the difference in stillbirths related to anomaly in boys and girls.

A3. H_0: There is no difference between the stillbirths related to anomaly in boys and girls.

The main point to remember is that χ^2 must not be calculated on rates, but on actual numbers.
The numbers of stillbirths can be calculated as:

$$(309\ 722 \times 1.23)10^{-3} = 381 \text{ (boys)}$$
$$(291\ 804 \times 2.29)10^{-3} = 669 \text{ (girls)}$$

If H_0 were valid, we would expect equal numbers of stillbirths in both groups, i.e. 525 per group.
Therefore:

$$\chi^2 = \frac{(381 - 525)^2}{525} + \frac{(669 - 525)^2}{525} = 79$$

From Appendix 2 we see that $P \ll 0.001$ for $\chi^2 = 79$ with 1 degree of freedom. We can thus reject the Null Hypothesis.

Q4. The table below shows the gestational age (GA) at amniocentesis of 517 patients. Mean GA was 18.67 weeks, with a standard deviation of 2.226 weeks. Using χ^2 demonstrate whether or not this data is normally-distributed.

Weeks GA	No. of patients
15	17
16	65
17	94
18	108
19	74
20	55
21	36
22	33
23	11
24	24

A4. H_0: The data follow a normal distribution
Use Equation 6 to calculate z for each weekly interval. Thus the

expected proportion of the normal distribution in the 15 week group is:

$$z = \frac{15 - 18.67}{2.226} = -1.65$$

From Appendix 1 we see that this covers the area 0.0495 or 4.95%. 4.95% of 517 is 25.6. We would thus expect 25.6 patients to have undergone amniocentesis at 15 weeks gestation if the data were normally-distributed. Having calculated all the expected values, χ^2 is calculated from Equation 11.

$$\chi^2 = 123.7$$

There are 10 groups in the table. There are therefore $(10 - 1 - 2 =) 7$ degrees of freedom. Appendix 2 shows that $\chi^2 = 123.7$ is highly statistically-significant, $p < 0.001$. We therefore reject the Null Hypothesis, and conclude that the data is not normally-distributed.

4

Simple significance tests

So far we have largely considered descriptive statistics. Also frequently used are comparative statistics in which we compare two samples in order to test whether or not they are likely to have come from the same population. Use your common sense about this. If you have two samples, each of more than 100 patients, and there is no overlap between the two ranges of the parameter studied, it is a waste of time formally to calculate the statistical significance of this difference. Comparative statistics are concerned with the grey areas in which sample ranges overlap, and the assessment of whether or not this degree of overlap indicates that both samples are from the same population.

This chapter considers some of the simpler ways of assessing the possible statistical significance of observed differences between groups of data in which a normal distribution is not assumed, or which has been assessed on other than interval scales, that is, non-parametric data.

Ranking tests
The various *ranking* tests are among the simplest forms of test for statistical significance of differences between groups and do not assume a knowledge of the underlying distribution of the data. They are also very useful for small samples. The simplest such test is probably *the sign test*.

Example 4.1
A pharmaceutical company wished to assess whether one shape of tablet was easier for patients to swallow than another. Ten patients were asked to swallow tablets of both shape A and shape B in random order. Their preferences are summarized in Table 4.1, '+' indicating the shape found easier to swallow by each patient.

The simplest, albeit least sensitive, test of this hypothesis involves the use of the table in Appendix 3, which is simplicity itself. In this example we see that 9 of 10 patients found tablet shape A easier

Table 4.1

Patient	Shape A	Shape B
1	+	−
2	+	−
3	+	−
4	+	−
5	+	−
6	+	−
7	+	−
8	+	−
9	−	+
10	+	−

H_0: Tablet shape does not influence ease of swallowing

to swallow than shape B, that is, there were 9 similar signs. Appendix 3 shows that, for $n = 10$ pairs, if only one sign differs, then the treatment (shape) is exerting a statistically-significant effect. If we had only had 8 patients, one of whom found shape B preferable, the result would not have been significant on this test.

With this kind of test, if you are studying a 'Yes; No; Don't know' situation, ignore the number of 'Don't knows'.

χ^2 again

Another way of dealing with such data is to use a χ^2 test as described in Chapter 3. This is shown here to illustrate the principle. Normally, of course, one would not use χ^2 when $n < 20$ (see p. 38). Given H_0, we would expect 5 patients to prefer shape A and 5 to prefer shape B. In this sample, 9 of the 10 patients preferred shape A.

From Equation 11:

$$\chi^2 = \frac{(9 - 5)^2}{5} + \frac{(1 - 5)^2}{5} = 6.4$$

Two points arise from this. The first is that, since squaring removes the effect of positive or negative sign, Equation 11 can be compressed *under circumstances such as these* to the form:

$$\chi^2 = \frac{(O_b - O_s)^2}{n} \qquad \text{Equation 12}$$

where O_b is the bigger, and O_s the smaller, observed value. Substituting data from Example 4.1 we calculate:

$$\chi^2 = \frac{(9 - 1)^2}{10} = 6.4$$

The second point is this. Appendix 2 shows a χ^2 of 6.4 with 1 degree of freedom to be significant, $P < 0.05$. *But*, the number in the sample is very small ($n = 10$). It is therefore usual to apply a correction factor, known as Yates's *correction for continuity* This is because the theory underlying the distribution of χ^2 is actually based on an assumption of continuity in data, whereas data on a ranking scale is not continuous. This departure from theory is most pronounced when sample sizes are small. The correction is very simply made by calculating χ^2 from:

$$\chi_Y^2 = \frac{[O_b - O_s) - 1]^2}{n} \qquad \text{Equation 13}$$

In the example above, we would calculate:

$$\chi_Y^2 = \frac{[(9 - 1) - 1]^2}{10} = \frac{49}{10} = 4.9$$

Appendix 2 shows that this is still significant, ($P < 0.05$). We therefore reject the Null Hypothesis.

The answer to the question: 'When do I use Yates's correction?' is that, as a general rule, it is safest *always* to apply it when n is less than 100. There is some discussion among statisticians as to whether its use is appropriate with larger samples.

This is an appropriate point at which to remind you of Type II errors, that is, of accepting a Null Hypothesis when it is, in reality, invalid (Chapter 1). This is most likely to occur when small sample sizes are used. If a statistical test produces a 'Not statistically significant' result when intuition tells you that there *is* a difference, increase the numbers in the sample. This is unlikely to alter the result if the Null Hypothesis is valid, but will frequently allow the unmasking of a statistically-significant effect.

Tests such as those above can also be used when a variable can be measured on an interval scale before and after treatment. If, for example, the blood pressure in a group of patients is measured before and after treatment with an antihypertensive agent, the results can simply be expressed as 'Lower/Not lower', rather than as mmHg, and a sign test or χ^2 test applied. This is useful for a quick check of data, or when data are skewed, but is not especially sensitive. If a situation arises in which the possible assessments are 'Better; Worse; Don't know', the numbers of 'Don't knows' are again ignored, and n in Equation 13 is the number 'Better' plus the number 'Worse'.

χ^2 and contingency tables.

We are frequently presented with qualitative, rather than quantitative, data taking the form 'Mild; Moderate; Severe' or 'Better; Worse; Unchanged' in relation to some other parameter which may or may not be capable of quantitative description. Potential effects of, say, treatment on outcome, can be assessed using a contingency table, as shown below.

Example 4.2
The manufacturers of an anti-depressant drug, A, produced a variant drug B which, they claimed, was more effective. A trial was established in which 240 patients were allocated at random to treatment with either drug A, drug B or a placebo. Patients were asked after treatment for one month whether they felt better, worse or no different. The data obtained are summarized in Table 4.2.

Table 4.2 Contingency table relating outcome of treatment to drug administered. Bold numerals denote the numbers expected from the Null Hypothesis.

Outcome	Drug A		Drug B		Drug P		Totals
Better	47		52		32		131
		44.8		**42.0**		**44.2**	
Unchanged	29		22		33		84
		28.7		**27.0**		**28.4**	
Worse	6		3		16		25
		8.5		**8.0**		**8.4**	
Totals	82		77		81		240

Our Null Hypothesis states that the treatment given does not influence the outcome. If this were so, then the number of patients receiving drug A who reported an improvement should relate both to the <u>proportion of the total number of patients given drug A, and to the</u> <u>proportion of the total number of patients who reported an</u> <u>improvement</u> in symptoms. We can thus calculate the expected number of patients in each cell of the table. So, for example, in the cell Drug A/Felt better we would expect to find $82 \times 131/240 = 44.8$ patients. The expected figures for each cell are shown in heavy type in Table 4.2. It is a good idea to check your calculation of the expected frequencies by confirming that the sum of the expected frequencies in each row or column is the same as the sum of the observed frequencies for that row or column. Thus in Table 4.2 both the total observed and the total expected in the column relating to drug A is 82. χ^2 can then be assessed as usual from Equation 11. Thus:

$$\chi^2 = \frac{(47 - 44.8)^2}{44.8} + \frac{(52 - 42)^2}{42} + \ldots + \frac{(16 - 8.4)^2}{8.4}$$

$$= 18.27$$

The number of degrees of freedom is given by multiplying the number of groups (columns) minus 1 by the number of rows minus 1. We subtract 1 in each instance, since once we know the numbers in two of the groups or rows and the total, we can calculate the third. In this instance we have $(3 - 1)(3 - 1) = 4$ degrees of freedom. From Appendix 2 we see that $P < 0.01$ for a χ^2 of 18.27 with 4 degrees of freedom. It therefore appears that there is a significant departure from the Null Hypothesis. Note that although this exercise shows us that there is an association between treatment and outcome, it tells us nothing more about that association. Inspection of observed and expected values tells us that the outcome is worse following treatment with the placebo, but is drug B more efficacious than drug A?

To assess this, one could compare the outcome with drugs A and B, excluding the placebo data.

Table 4.3 shows this comparison.

Table 4.3 Contingency table relating outcome of treatment to drug administered. Bold numerals denote the numbers expected from the Null Hypothesis.

Outcome	Drug A		Drug B		Totals
Better	47		52		99
		51.1		**47.9**	
Unchanged	29		22		51
		26.3		**24.7**	
Worse	6		3		9
		4.6		**4.4**	
Totals	82		77		159

Now $\chi^2 = 2.123$, with $(3 - 1)(2 - 1) = 2$ degrees of freedom, which Appendix 2 shows not to be significant. We can therefore accept the Null Hypothesis that there was no difference between the effects of the two drugs, and reject the manufacturer's claim.

It will be seen in Table 4.3, that in fact the expected number in two cells is less than 5, which, you will remember, should not be the case for χ^2. It is often possible to overcome such a difficulty by *collapsing* groups or rows. Thus we could say that we are only interested in whether the patient felt better or not, and collapse the 'Unchanged' and 'Worse' categories (Table 4.4).

Table 4.4 Contingency table of the data in Table 4.3, collapsing categories 'Unchanged' and 'Worse'

Outcome	Drug A		Drug B		Totals
Better	47		52		99
		51.1		47.9	
No better	35		25		60
		30.9		29.1	
Totals	82		77		159

χ^2 is then 1.801, with 1 degree of freedom, supporting the Null Hypothesis.

2 × 2 contingency tables

Tables such as Table 4.4 with two groups (columns) and 2 rows occur very commonly, and lend themselves to a quick method of analysis. Table 4.5 represents a 2 × 2 table symbolically.

Table 4.5 A general 2 × 2 contingency table

	Drug	Placebo	
Improved	a	b	$a + b$
Not improved	c	d	$c + d$
	$a + c$	$b + d$	n

χ^2 for such a table can be calculated from:

$$\chi^2 = \frac{n(ad - bc)^2}{(a+b)(c+d)(a+c)(b+d)}$$ Equation 14

However, since it frequently happens that the numbers studied are fairly small, it is advisable to apply a correction for continuity, as previously described. Doing this gives us:

$$\chi^2 = \frac{n[(ad-bc) - \frac{1}{2}n]^2}{(a+b)(c+d)(a+c)(b+d)}$$ Equation 15

If we substitute the data from Table 4.4 in Equation 15 we calculate.

$$\chi^2 = \frac{159[(47 \times 25) - (52 \times 35) - 79.5]^2}{(47 + 52)(35 + 25)(47 + 82)(52 + 77)}$$

$$= 1.355$$

Again, there is only $(2 - 1)(2 - 1) = 1$ degree of freedom. This approximation is quick and easy to do and should be used when there are only 2 columns and 2 rows provided that sample size is reasonably large, so that were you to calculate the expected frequencies, none would be less than 5.

Fisher's exact test

We have already seen that if the expected frequency in any cell of a proposed χ^2 contingency table is less than 5, χ^2 should not be used. Sometimes however we only have data from a very small series, perhaps when studying a very rare disease, and we wish to be able to make some statement about, say, the efficacy of two treatments. Under these circumstances, Fisher's exact test is used which is a specialized form of a 2×2 table. This can also be useful when the numbers in either the rows or columns have been previously fixed, as, for example, by allocating 10 patients to group 1 and 10 to group 2.

Example 4.3

In an early trial of the effect of cytotoxic drugs on the outcome of patients suffering from stage 3B Hodgkin's disease, data was available from 7 patients who received chemotherapy as part of their treatment, and 9 who did not. Six of the seven patients so treated were alive at 2 years after diagnosis, whereas only 2 of the 9 were. Was chemotherapy treatment associated with a significant improvement in prognosis?

H_0: There is no difference in outcome with treatment

Fisher's exact test in effect assesses all possible outcomes of treatment with and without chemotherapy and allows us to assess the probability of the outcome we actually observed having arisen if the Null Hypothesis is valid. We therefore need to calculate the probability of obtaining our observed result, or any more extreme result. This is done by first calculating:

$$P_1 = \frac{(a+b)!\,(c+d)!\,(a+c)!\,(b+d)!}{n!\,a!\,b!\,c!\,d!} \qquad \text{Equation 16}$$

using the symbols a, b, c and d as in the cells of the 2×2 contingency table in Table 4.5. The exclamation mark ! simply means 'factorial'. Thus 5! is shorthand for $5 \times 4 \times 3 \times 2 \times 1$. Both 1! and 0! equal 1.

Table 4.6 summarises the data of Example 4.3.

Substituting in Equation 16 gives:

$$P_1 = \frac{8!\,8!\,7!\,9!}{16!\,6!\,2!\,1!\,7!}$$

$$= \frac{40320 \times 40320 \times 5040 \times 362\,880}{(2.092 \times 10^{13}) \times 720 \times 2 \times 1 \times 5040}$$

$$= 0.0195$$

Table 4.6 The 2-year survival of 16 patients with stage 3B Hodgkin's disease by treatment with or without chemotherapy

Treatment Outcome	+ Cytotoxics	− Cytotoxics	Totals
Alive	6	2	8
Dead	1	7	8
Totals	7	9	16

To calculate the more extreme probabilities, reduce the smallest number in any of the cells by 1, while holding the totals constant. Table 4.6 then becomes:

Treatment Outcome	+ Cytotoxics	− Cytotoxics	Totals
Alive	7	1	8
Dead	0	8	8
Totals	7	9	16

The more extreme probabilities (P_2) are also calculated from Equation 16:

$$P_2 = \frac{8! \, 8! \, 7! \, 9!}{16! \, 7! \, 1! \, 0! \, 8!}$$

$$= \frac{40320 \times 40320 \times 5040 \times 362\,880}{(2.092 \times 10^{13}) \times 5040 \times 1 \times 1 \times 40320}$$

$$= 0.0007$$

The total $P_1 + P_2 = 0.0202$, which is the probability of finding the observed distribution of data, or a more extreme one. If treatment with cytotoxic drugs could not be expected to be associated with a worse outcome than other treatment alone, then we would only be interested in one 'tail' of the possible distribution, and we would reject H_0, $P < 0.02$. Cytotoxic drugs are, however, potentially harmful in themselves, so in this instance we are interested in both 'tails' of the possible distribution. The approximate measure of this is given by $(P_1 + P_2) \times 2$, which in the example above would give a 'two-tailed' P of 0.04. We would thus still reject H_0, and conclude that, in this small series, treatment with chemotherapy was associated with a better outcome. The concept of a one-tailed test is further discussed in Chapter 5.

Wilcoxon's signed rank test
This is a slightly more sensitive way of comparing, for example, treatment groups.

Example 4.4
Nine pairs of sex-matched sibling rats were used in a study of the effect of a dietary supplement on body-weight. One of each pair was given the supplement each day for two weeks while the other received a placebo. Table 4.7 shows the *difference* in weight between the supplemented and unsupplemented members of each pair at the end of this time. <u>Was the administration of the supplement associated with a significant change in weight?</u>

Table 4.7   The differential effect of dietary supplementation on body weight in rats

Pair	Difference (g)	Rank
1	+3	4.5
2	+8	7
3	+10	8
4	-1	(−) 1
5	+2	3
6	-1.5	(−) 2
7	+5	6
8	+3	4.5
9	+11	9

H_0: The dietary supplement had no significant effect on weight.

If this hypothesis were correct, then there would be an approximately equal number of negative and positive differences, so that the total ranks for negative and positive would be approximately the same. What we try to do is to assess how far our observations depart from this hypothetical result.

The first thing to do is to rank the differences, ignoring the sign (+ or −) and ranking the smallest as 1. Note that where two differences are identical, they are each given the *average* of the next two ranks. In the example above, there were two differences of 3 g which happened both to be positive, although the sign doesn't matter for this. The first three ranks have already been assigned, so the next two are 4 and 5. The average rank, 4.5, is therefore given to *both* 3 g differences, and the next biggest difference ranks 6.

When all differences have been ranked, the signs are restored. Add up the ranks for the smaller-sized group, in this case those with the negative sign. The total of these ranks, $T = 1 + 2 = 3$. This number is then looked up in a table of rank sums such as Appendix 4. For nine pairs, T must be 5 or less for significance at the 5% level. Since $T = 3$, $P < 0.05$ and the Null Hypothesis can be rejected. Of course, sometimes when this test is performed, the smaller-*sized* group will have the higher ranks. In this instance, the rank total must be equal to or greater than the larger of the two numbers shown in Appendix 4.

It is sensible at this point to consider just what we mean by 'paired data'. In Example 4.4, pairs of sex-matched, sibling rats were used to assess the effect of a dietary supplement on growth rate. They were matched for sex, because of known differing growth rates with gender, and were siblings to allow for any intra-uterine factors which might subsequently affect growth rate, and which could differ from litter to litter. Provided that the supplemented and unsupplemented groups were kept under otherwise identical conditions, the experimenter could fairly assume that any change in growth rate was related to the effect of dietary supplementation. Even so, however, there will be some genetic variation between the rats, and although we hope that this will balance out in the treated and untreated groups, it introduces an element of uncertainty.

The optimum pairing occurs when a patient or subject can act as their own control. For example, the one-minute forced expiratory volume (FEV_1) can be measured in an asthmatic patient before and after the administration of a β_2 agonist and the change in FEV_1 noted. Under these circumstances there is only one variable to consider, allowing greater confidence to be placed in the results.

There are however some circumstances under which it is not possible to use a patient as his or her own control, as, for example, in an investigation of whether a particular chronic disease is associated with changes in some specific parameter. What may be done under these circumstances is to 'match' each patient in the disease group with another patient similar in as many respects as possible to the study patient, but without the disease. The variables which must be matched must take into account the nature of the disease and any factor known to influence it. Inevitably though, these will be far from perfect matches, and a number of non-parametric statistical tests exist to assess the significance of differences between groups of *unpaired* data.

Wilcoxon's ranking test for unpaired data (Mann-Whitney test)

Example 4.5
Table 4.8 shows blood glucose concentrations ($mmol \cdot l^{-1}$) 2 hours after ingestion of 50 g glucose in water in 10 women with known diabetes mellitus and 8 patients with previous gestational diabetes.

Does the 2 hour blood glucose (BG) concentration differ between the two groups?

Table 4.8

	Diabetic		Gestational diabetes	
BG	Rank		BG	Rank
11	13.5		6	2
9	7		10	10.5
11	13.5		8	4
10	10.5		5	1
10	10.5		9	7
15	17.5		8	4
12	15.5		12	15.5
10	10.5		8	4
9	7			
15	17.5			
Total	123			48

H_0: The 2 h blood glucose concentration does not differ significantly in the two groups.

If H_0 is tenable, we would expect the data in the two samples to have been drawn from the same population. This may be easier to visualise in terms of distribution curves. The Null Hypothesis supposes that the blood glucose concentrations in the two groups come from a single population, as shown in Figure 4.1 (broken curve). If, in fact, there are two populations there will be two distribution curves (Fig. 4.1; solid curves). What the ranking tests measure is the degree of overlap (shaded) between the two. If this is small, T will be small for one group because the majority of its ranks will be in the left hand distribution, and it is probable that the samples come from different populations. Incidentally, although the hypothetical populations are shown as being approximately normally distributed in Figure 4.1 this is not a requirement for the test, since it is a nonparametric test.

The probability of the samples having come from the same population is tested by assigning ranks to all the blood glucose concentrations as though they were all part of one sample. Thus, although the five lowest blood glucose concentrations occur in the group with gestational diabetes, concentrations of 9 mmol $\cdot$ l^{-1} occur in both the diabetic and the gestational diabetic group, and are assigned their appropriate rank *in the total*. Note that when the same value occurs more than once, each is given the average value of the

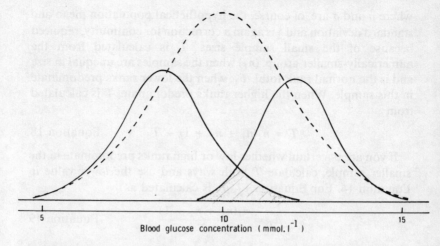

Blood glucose concentration (mmol. l^{-1})

Fig. 4.1 The broken curve (---) is the hypothetical population, as specified in the Null Hypothesis, from which both samples, (shown as solid curves) would be expected to have been drawn. If the degree of overlap (shaded) is less than a specified amount, then the Null Hypothesis can be rejected.

appropriate range of ranks. Thus a 2 h blood glucose concentration of 8 mmol · l^{-1} was found in three patients. Ranks 1 and 2 were already assigned so that these three patients covered ranks 3, 4 and 5; they were accordingly all assigned to rank 4. The next highest concentration, 9 mmol · l^{-1}, was also found in three patients, who thus covered ranks 6, 7 and 8. All were therefore assigned to rank 7. Check at the end that your last rank is indeed equal to $n_1 + n_2$ (18 in this example).

Once all values have been ranked the total ranks (T_1) in the numerically-smaller group (n_1) is calculated, and T_1 is looked up in Appendix 5. We see that for $n_1 = 8$ and n_2 (the number in the larger group) = 10, a T_1 of less than 53 indicates significance at the 5% level. We therefore reject H_0. We could also have done so had the total ranks in the smaller group exceeded 99.

You will see that Appendix 5 only related to sample sizes up to 19 and 14. When your sample sizes are larger than this it is reasonable to calculate a z value (Chapter 2) and use the table of the normal distribution (Appendix 1) to give the probability of the samples concerned having come from the same population. To do this, calculate:

$$z_T = \frac{(\mu_T - T - \frac{1}{2})}{\sigma_T}$$

Equation 17

where μ and σ are, of course, the hypothetical population mean and standard deviation and $\frac{1}{2}$ is again a correction for continuity, required because of the small sample sizes. T is calculated from the numerically-smaller group, (n_1) when the samples are unequal in size and is the normal rank total, T_1, when the lower ranks predominate in this sample. When the higher ranks predominate, T is calculated from

$$T = n_1(n_1 + n_2 + 1) - T_1 \qquad \text{Equation 18}$$

If you are uncertain whether low or high ranks predominate in the smaller sample, calculate T both ways and use the *lower* value in Equation 14. For Equation 17, μ_T is calculated as:

$$\mu_T = \frac{n_1(n_1 + n_2 + 1)}{2} \qquad \text{Equation 19}$$

and σ_T as:

$$\sigma_T = \sqrt{\frac{n_2\mu}{6}} \qquad \text{Equation 20}$$

Example 4.6
To illustrate this, imagine that the sample sizes in Example 4.5 were increased to 20 and 18 respectively, and that T_1 for the gestational diabetic group was 243. Then:

$$\mu_T = \frac{18(18 + 20 + 1)}{2} = 351$$

and

$$\sigma_T = \sqrt{\frac{20 \times 351}{6}} = 34.21$$

and

$$z_T = \frac{(351 - 243 - \frac{1}{2})}{34.21} = 3.142$$

Consulting Appendix 1, we see that for $z = 3.142$, less than 0.1% of the total area will lie in the "tail" beyond z. *But* we have no *a priori* reason for thinking that we should be considering only 1 tail of the distribution. We therefore have to consider *both* tails of the distribution, so that $P < 0.002$ rather than $P < 0.001$.

SUMMARY OF CHAPTER 4

1. *All* significance tests are designed to assess the probability of the observed result having arisen if the Null Hypothesis is valid. By convention, if the result will have arisen less than one in twenty times, if the Null Hypothesis is valid, the result is said to be statistically significant, $P < 0.05$, and the Null Hypothesis is rejected.

2. Whenever the effect of a treatment or procedure can be summarized on a 'plus or minus' scale (e.g. 'better/worse'; 'more/less') a *sign test* can be used to assess the statistical significance of the results. To do this, simply count the number of like signs ($+$ or $-$) which occur less often, and refer this number to Appendix 3 in relation to your total number of pairs. When there is a 'Don't know' or 'Unchanged' category, omit that data from your calculation. This is a very quick, but not a very sensitive test.

3. A χ^2 *test* (Equation 12; Appendix 2) can also be used to test data of this kind. It is usual to apply Yates's correction for continuity (Equation 13) for samples in which $n < 100$.

4. *Contingency tables* (e.g. Table 4.2) can be drawn up and used to assess whether two or more procedures are exerting a significant effect on two or more groups. This again makes use of the χ^2 statistic to assess whether the data fit the pattern predicted on the Null Hypothesis (no effect) or not. If the expected value in any cell of the table is less than 5, two appropriate groups should be run together (collapsed) to overcome this. There are $(g - 1)(r - 1)$ degrees of freedom, where g = number of groups and r = number of rows in the table.

5. In the special instance of a contingency table with two rows and two groups (columns), χ^2 can be quickly calculated from Equation 15 and referred to Appendix 2 with 1 degree of freedom.

6. When very small numbers are unavoidable, *Fisher's exact test* may be used, which is a specialized example of a 2×2 table. P is calculated directly from Equation 16.

7. Where *ranks* can be assigned to changes in *paired* data, the *Wilcoxon signed rank test* is used. Ranks are assigned to the differences between paired observations, regardless of whether the differences are positive ($+$) or negative ($-$). The $+$ and $-$ signs are then restored to the pairs, and the sum of ranks (T) for the numerically smaller group (by sign) is calculated. T is then referred to Appendix 4.

8. Where data can be ranked but arises from two different groups of observations, rather than from paired observations, a variant on

the Wilcoxon rank sum test, also known as the Mann-Whitney test, is used. Ranks are assigned to the data as though it all arose from one sample. The ranks in the numerically smaller group are then added up and referred to Appendix 5. Appendix 5 relates only to sample sizes up to $n_1 = 19$ and $n_2 = 14$. When the sample sizes are bigger than this, calculate z from Equation 17 and refer it to Appendix 1 as usual.

QUESTIONS FOR CHAPTER 4

Q1. The effect of an antihypertensive agent alone on diastolic blood pressure was assessed in ten patients. When a diuretic was added to the treatment regime, the fall in blood pressure was found to be as summarized below. Was the diuretic significantly changing control of blood pressure?

Change in
fall in BP: $+2$ 0 -1 $+3$ $+5$ $+4$ $+2$ $+5$ $+1$ $+2$

H_0: The addition of a diuretic was not associated with a change in the fall in diastolic pressure.

A1. *Sign test*: There was no difference from the mean overall fall in blood pressure in one patient; we thus have nine patients to consider. Eight showed greater falls than the mean; one showed a lesser fall. Appendix 3 shows this not to be significant.

Wilcoxon rank sum: When the resultant differences are ranked, ignoring the zero, we find that the smallest difference, 1, occurs with both a $+$ and a $-$ sign. Its rank is thus 1.5. Appendix 4 shows us that for 9 patients, a total rank of 1.5 will occur in less than one such sample in 50 were the Null Hypothesis to hold. We therefore reject H_0, $P < 0.02$. This is an example of the greater sensitivity of a Rank Sum test than a Sign test.

Q2. Haemoglobin concentration was measured in nine Asian women and nine Caucasians at an antenatal clinic. The values found were:

Asian: 7.3, 8.4, 8.2, 9.7, 10.2, 8.7, 9.1, 8.9, 9.4

Caucasian: 8.5, 9.8, 9.4, 11.4, 10.7, 9.9, 10.1, 9.6, 10.0

Do these data suggest that there is a difference in haemoglobin concentration with ethnic group?

A2. H_0: Haemoglobin concentration does not differ significantly in the two groups

First, rank the haemoglobin measurements as though they were all from the same sample.

Asian: 7.3, 8.4, 8.2, 9.7, 10.2, 8.7, 9.1, 8.9, 9.4
           1   **3**   **2**   **11**   **16**   **5**   **7**   **6**   **8.5**

Caucasian: 10.0, 9.8, 9.4, 11.4, 10.7, 9.9, 10.1, 9.6, 8.5
           14   **12**   **8.5** ·**18**   **17**   **13**   **15**   **10**   **4**

Then add up the ranks in either group; since they are equal in size it does not matter which you sum.

$$T_{Asian} = 59.5$$
$$T_{Caucasian} = 111.5$$

From Appendix 5 we see that when $n_1 = 9$ and $n_2 = 9$ T must be either less than 62 or greater than 109. T_{Asian} is less than 62 and $T_{Caucasian}$ is greater than 109; either T would therefore have given us the answer that there is less than one chance in 20 ($P < 0.05$) of these two samples having been taken from the same population.

Q3. 14 patients were seen in 6 months in an Accident and Emergency department following concussion associated with a riding accident. Four patients were found to have fractured skulls, none of whom had been wearing protective headgear. Only one of the 10 patients who had been wearing a riding cap suffered a fractured skull. Did the wearing of protective headgear afford a significant degree of protection?

A3. This is a very small sample of patients; it is therefore appropriate to use Fisher's exact test, *not* a χ^2 test.

H_0: The wearing of a riding cap did not afford a significant degree of protection.

$$P_1 = \frac{9! \, 5! \, 10! \, 4!}{14! \, 9! \, 0! \, 1! \, 4!}$$

$$= \frac{362\,880 \times 120 \times 3\,628\,800 \times 24}{(8.717 \times 10^{10}) \times 362\,880 \times 1 \times 24}$$

$$= 0.005$$

Since one of the cells already has a zero entry, P_2 cannot be calculated and $p = 0.005$ is the total probability of this outcome having arisen if the Null Hypothesis were valid. There is no theoretical reason to suppose that the wearing of a riding cap will *increase* the likelihood of suffering a fractured skull. We therefore propose a one-tailed test and reject the Null Hypothesis, $P = 0.005$.

Q4. A sample of 400 consecutive patients presenting at an allergy clinic were randomly allocated to treatment with either a long-established antihistamine (192 patients) or with a new type of drug (208 patients). When they were seen again, 80.2% of the patients receiving the established antihistamine reported an improvement in symptoms, while 87.5% of those given the new drug had obtained symptomatic relief. Was there a significant difference between the effect of the two drugs?

A4. This kind of data lends itself well to a χ^2 test *but* you must remember to convert the percentages to actual numbers first.

H_0: The two drugs were equally effective

80.2% of 192 is 154 patients, and 87.5% of 208 is 182 patients. We use a 2×2 contingency table since there are 2 columns (groups): 'Old drug' and 'New drug' and 2 rows: 'Better' and 'Not better'.

	Old drug	New drug	Totals
Better	154	182	336
Not Better	38	26	64
Totals	192	208	400

Substituting in Equation 14 gives us:

$$\chi^2 = \frac{400\left[(154 \times 26) - (182 \times 38)\right]^2}{336 \times 64 \times 208 \times 192}$$

$$= 3.949$$

Appendix 2 shows us that with 1 degree of freedom, a χ^2 of 3.949 is significant, $P < 0.05$. We therefore reject the Null Hypothesis.

Q5. Eight patients were each given 2 different analgesics, A and B, in a cross-over trial of pain relief. Seven considered pain relief to be greater with analgesic A. Is this difference statistically-significant?

A5. H_0: There was no difference in perceived pain relief in response to the two analgesics

$$\chi_Y^2 = \frac{\left[(O_b - O_s) - 1\right]^2}{n} = \frac{\left[(7 - 1) - 1\right]^2}{8}$$

$$= 3.125$$

Appendix 2 shows this not to be significant, and we thus reject the Null Hypothesis. However, the numbers concerned are very small, and this could well be an example of a Type II error. Intuition suggests enlarging the trial.

Q6. The trial of analgesics A and B in the question above was enlarged to cover eighty patients, of whom seventy found greater pain relief with analgesic A. Is this difference statistically significant?

A6. H_0: There was no difference in perceived pain relief in response to the two analgesics

$$\chi_Y^2 = \frac{[(70 - 10) - 1]^2}{80} = \frac{59^2}{80}$$

$$= 43.51$$

We see from Appendix 2 that a χ^2 of this magnitude is statistically very highly significant, $P \ll 0.001$. With such a sample size we can confidently reject the Null Hypothesis.

Q7. A study of the effects of amniocentesis on the subsequent incidence of threatened premature delivery was carried out in 289 women with carefully matched controls. 35 women who underwent amniocentesis subsequently threatened to go into labour before 37 weeks gestation, while only 10 control patients did so. Was amniocentesis associated with an increased likelihood of premature labour?

A7. H_0: Amniocentesis was not associated with an altered risk of premature labour

Tabulate the data for ease of scrutiny.

Premature labour	Amniocentesis No	Yes	Totals
No	279 **266.5**	254 **266.5**	533
Yes	10 **22.5**	35 **22.5**	45
Total	289	289	578

χ^2 is an appropriate statistic to calculate here. This can be done using either Equation 11 or Equation 14. It is instructive to calculate it both ways, to satisfy yourself that, under the special circumstances of a 2 × 2 contingency table, these two equations give the same answer.

χ^2 here is 15.06 which, with 1 degree of freedom, is highly significant, $P < 0.001$. We thus reject the Null Hypothesis and suggest that amniocentesis is associated with a greater incidence of threatened premature delivery.

Q8. In a comparison of a new rapid laboratory method for measuring serum osmolality with an older one, the osmolality $(mmol \cdot kg^{-1})$ in 13 samples was determined by both methods. The new method gave results which differed from the old as described below. Was there a consistent difference between the two methods?

New: 283 280 278 281 297 289 277 280 284 276 290 279 282
Old: 282 280 275 279 294 288 277 281 282 277 286 276 283

A8. H_0: There was no difference in serum osmolality when measured by these two methods

The simplest test is the sign test. Inspection of the data shows that, ignoring the zeros, there were 8 positive and 3 negative differences. Appendix 3 shows that, to achieve statistical significance with $n = 11$ pairs, 10 of the differences need to be of the same sign. We thus accept the Null Hypothesis.

However, the sign test is not very sensitive, and inspection of the data does suggest that there may indeed be a practical difference between the two methods. The Wilcoxon rank sum test is a more sensitive test for this kind of data, so calculate the difference in osmolality for each sample and rank them, ignoring both the zeros and whether the difference is positive or negative. When the signs are restored, T for the numerically-smaller group, in this example those 3 in which the old method read higher than the new, is calculated as:

$$T = 9$$

Appendix 4 shows that, for $n = 11$ (because you have omitted the zeros) T should be $\leqslant 13$ or $\geqslant 53$ for any difference to be statistically significant. We thus reject the Null Hypothesis: $P < 0.05$.

5

More simple significance tests

In Chapter 4 we considered some of the simpler ways of assessing the possible significance of observed differences between groups of data in which a normal distribution was not assumed, or which had been assessed on non-interval scales. Frequently however data is given on an interval scale, and broadly conforms to a normal distribution. This kind of data lends itself to more sensitive testing of departures from a Null Hypothesis.

Large samples ($n > 30$)
Consider first of all the comparison of a sample with a known population mean. Our Null Hypothesis of course states that the sample mean does not differ significantly from the population mean. We have already seen in Chapter 2 that the standard error of a sample mean tells us how closely that sample mean approximates to the population mean *from which that sample is drawn*. We can therefore calculate the ratio between the *difference* between our sample mean and the population mean, and the standard error of our sample. Thus:

$$z = \frac{\bar{x} - \mu}{s/\sqrt{n}}$$
                                                            Equation 21

This is, of course, very similar in format to Equation 6. We then use Appendix 1 to assess the probability of this ratio having occurred if the sample came from the normal population. In other words, we are testing whether our sample mean is more than ± 1.96 standard errors from the hypothetical population mean.

Example 5.1
The mean plasma cortisol concentration of healthy, non-stressed subjects at 9 a.m. is 450 nmol $\cdot$ l^{-1} with a range of 150–700 nmol $\cdot$ l^{-1}. Plasma cortisol concentration under similar conditions in a group of 33 patients with Cushing's syndrome was 1150 nmol $\cdot$ l^{-1} with a

standard deviation of $300\,nmol \cdot l^{-1}$. Is this difference statistically-significant?

H_0: There is no difference between the normal population mean and the mean value in patients with Cushing's syndrome

We can calculate z from Equation 21 as:

$$z = \frac{1150-450}{300/\sqrt{33}} = 13.40$$

Appendix 1 shows us that for a z of 13.4, the probability is much less than 1 in 10 000 of the sample having come from the normal population. We reject the Null Hypothesis, and state confidently that patients with Cushing's syndrome studied under these circumstances have substantially higher mean plasma cortisol concentrations than normal patients.

In this example, the difference between $\bar{x}$ and μ gave a positive answer, and thus a positive z. It can, of course, also be the case that $\bar{x}$ is bigger than μ, resulting in a negative z. This makes *no difference* to how you use Appendix 1, since the negative and positive ends of the z distribution are mirror-images of each other. This is also true for 't' tables (see below).

This kind of calculation of course depends on our knowing the population mean. It is much more usual not to know the true population mean. We often wish to assess whether data from two samples whose mean and standard deviation we can calculate have each come from the same population. Again, we use the standard error about the sample means to tell us the probability of those two samples having been taken from the same population.

What we effectively do is to assess the *mean difference* between the two samples and calculate a 'combined' standard error. If the ratio between the *difference* between the two sample means and their combined standard error is more than 1.96 we can say that the probability of our having drawn two such samples from the same population is less than 1 in 20 ($P < 0.05$). Again, Appendix 1 is used to assess the degree of significance. These calculations should only be done when the number in each sample is greater than 30.

The required ratio is calculated as:

$$z = \frac{\bar{x}_1 - \bar{x}_2}{\sqrt{\dfrac{s_1^2}{n_1} + \dfrac{s_2^2}{n_2}}} \qquad \text{Equation 22}$$

where $\bar{x}_1$ = mean of the 1st sample

$\bar{x}_2$ = mean of the 2nd sample

s_1^2 = variance of the 1st sample

s_2^2 = variance of the 2nd sample

n_1 = number in the 1st sample

n_2 = number in the 2nd sample

and remembering that $\sqrt{s^2/n}$ is simply an alternative way of calculating the standard error (Equation 8).

Example 5.2
The mean plasma volume at term in 32 women in their first pregnancy was 3.7 l, standard deviation 0.62 l. In their second pregnancy, the mean plasma volume at term was 4.2 l, standard deviation 0.6 l. Is this difference statistically significant?

H_0: The observed difference in plasma volume is not statistically significant

First, calculate the 'combined standard error' (SE_c):

$$SE_c = \sqrt{\frac{0.62^2}{32} + \frac{0.6^2}{32}} = 0.153$$

The difference in plasma volume between the two parity groups is $(3.7 - 4.2 =) - 0.5$ l. Thus:

$$z = -\frac{0.5}{0.153} = -3.268$$

Reference to Appendix 1 shows us that there is less than 1 chance in 500 ($P < 0.002$ with a 2-tailed test, p. 76) of such a ratio being obtained if both samples had come from the same population. We thus reject the Null Hypothesis, and accept that, on this data, there is a greater plasma volume in second than in first pregnancies.

The comparison of two percentages (n in each group > 30).
We sometimes collect data which, although they logically follow a binomial distribution, are sufficiently numerous to let us use the normal distribution in assessing potential differences between two data sets.

The necessary calculations can be summarized as:

$$z = \frac{p_1 - p_2}{\sqrt{\dfrac{p \times (1 - p)}{n_1} + \dfrac{p \times (1 - p)}{n_2}}}$$ Equation 23

where p is the *overall* proportion of 'successes' or 'failures', p_1 and p_2 are the proportions of 'successes' or 'failures' in the two groups under investigation and n_1 and n_2 are the numbers in the two groups.

Example 5.3

Suppose, for example, that we want to compare the birth-rates in two groups each of 12 pregnant rabbits, one group having been given a daily dose of an antihypertensive drug under test, while the other was given a placebo. 93 baby rabbits were born to the does receiving the experimental drug, of which 22 were stillborn. 97 baby rabbits were born in the control group, of which 9 were stillborn. Was the administration of the drug associated with a significant change in the stillbirth rate?

H_0: Administration of the drug was not associated with a change in stillbirth rate

The stillbirth rates in the two groups are calculated as:

Experimental: $\dfrac{22}{93} = 0.237 \ (p_1)$

Control: $\dfrac{9}{97} = 0.093 \ (p_2)$

However, if H_0 is tenable, both samples will have come from a common population, of which the mean stillbirth rate (p) will be approximated by:

$$\frac{\text{total number stillborn}}{\text{total births}} = \frac{22 + 9}{93 + 97}$$

$$= 0.163, \text{ or } 16.3 \text{ per hundred births}$$

To calculate the variance of each stillbirth rate, we use Equation 10, since we have here a straightforward instance of 'proportion alive, p' and 'proportion dead, $1 - p$', that is, a binomial distribution. Thus:

$$s_p^2 = \frac{p \times (1 - p)}{n}$$

So for the treated group,

$$s_p^2 = \frac{0.163 \times (1 - 0.163)}{93} = 0.00147$$

and for the control group

$$s_p^2 = \frac{0.163 \times (1 - 0.163)}{97} = 0.00141$$

The sum of these two variances then gives us the variance of the difference between the two stillbirth rates. This combined variance = $(0.00147 + 0.00141 =)$ 0.00288, so that the combined standard deviation is 0.054. The ratio of the difference between the two stillbirth rates $(0.237 - 0.093 =)$ 0.144 to the combined standard deviation is thus:

$$z = 0.144/0.054 = 2.67$$

We see from Appendix 1 that the probability of obtaining such a ratio if both samples had come from the same population is less than 1 in 100. We can therefore say that administration of the test drug was associated with a significantly greater stillbirth rate, $P < 0.01$.

As noted in Chapter 3, the smaller p (or $1 - p$) is, then the bigger each n should be to allow valid use of this test.

Small samples—either or both $n \leqslant 30$

Unpaired data. As a rule of thumb, it is safe to say that if there is an overlap in the range covered by the smaller of two means plus its standard error, and the larger of the two means minus its standard error, then the two samples have been drawn from the same population and are not statistically significantly different. You therefore need not bother to do any further calculations. For example, if the bodyweights of 2 groups of patients are 67.0 ± 3.2 kg and 72.5 ± 3.5 kg, the values described above are 70.2 and 69 kg and the mean values will not be significantly different.

If there is no overlap, then we need to assess the probability of the samples having come from the same population. Because of the observed effect of n on the standard error (Chapter 2), we have to use a modification of the 'z' test for small samples, known as 'Student's t test'. We also have to ensure that the variances of the two samples are not grossly different from each other. For example, simple logic tells us that we should be careful when attempting to compare the two samples in Figure 5.1, because the distribution curves, although both approximately normal, are different. To put a numerical value on this logical reasoning, we simply calculate the ratio between the two variances, always putting the smaller as the divisor. The *variance ratio* (F) is thus:

$$F = \frac{s_1^2}{s_2^2} \qquad \text{Equation 24}$$

where s_1^2 = the bigger variance

s_2^2 = the smaller variance

This is known as an _F_-test, the abbreviation for 'Fisher's test', and should _always_ be performed before using a '_t_' test. The derived value is then looked up in tables of _F_, such as Appendix 6 with $[n_1 - 1]$ degrees of freedom on the horizontal axis and $[n_2 - 1]$ on the vertical axis, where n_1 is the number in the sample with the larger variance.

This very simple test is the basis for all _analysis of variance_. This is considered widely in standard statistical textbooks and in brief outline in Chapter 6.

If an _F_ test is significant, then _either_ use non-parametric tests (Chapter 4) _or_ use the modified '_z_' described later. _Do not_ use an ordinary '_t_' test.

If _F_ is not significant, then do a '_t_' test. This is expressed as:

$$t = \frac{\bar{x}_1 - \bar{x}_2}{s_c \sqrt{\dfrac{1}{n_1} + \dfrac{1}{n_2}}}$$
Equation 25

where s_c = 'combined standard deviation' of the two samples.

Do _not_ simply calculate the average standard deviation, but use:

$$s_c^2 = \frac{\Sigma_1(x - \bar{x}_1)^2 + \Sigma_2(x - \bar{x}_2)^2}{n_1 + n_2 - 2}$$
Equation 26

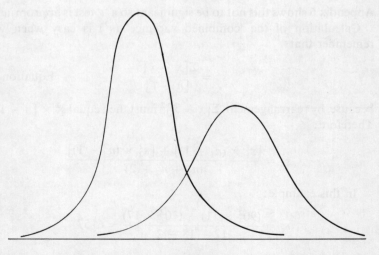

Fig. 5.1 Two distribution curves for sample data, not only with different means, but also with different variances

The similarities between Equations 22 and 25 are obvious. Again, the ratio between the differences between the means $[\bar{x}_1 - \bar{x}_2]$ and an estimate of 'combined standard error' is calculated. This ratio, t is then referred to a table of t values (Appendix 7).

Example 5.3
Data is summarized below from a survey of serum creatine kinase activity (CKA) in 12 marathon runners in training, and in 18 healthy subjects taking no more than one hour's mild to moderate exercise per day. Do these data suggest a change in basal CKA in subjects undertaking strenuous daily exercise?

	Mean CKA $(u \cdot l^{-1})$	s	n
Marathon runners	165	90	12
Others	100	70	18

H_0: CKA was not changed in subjects taking regular, hard exercise

First do an F test:

$$F = \frac{90^2}{70^2} = 1.65$$

Appendix 6 shows this not to be significant so a 't' test is appropriate.
Calculation of the 'combined variance' (s^2) is easy when we remember that:

$$s^2 = \frac{\Sigma[x - \bar{x}]^2}{[n - 1]}$$ Equation 4

because, by rearrangement, $\Sigma[x - \bar{x}]^2$ must then equal $s^2 \times [n - 1]$. Therefore:

$$s^2 = \frac{[s_1^2 \times (n_1 - 1)] + [s_2^2 \times (n^2 - 1)]}{(n_1 + n_2 - 2)}$$

In this example:

$$s_c^2 = \frac{(90^2 \times 11) + (70^2 \times 17)}{12 + 18 - 2} = 6157$$

so

$$s_c = \sqrt{6157} = 78.5$$

Substituting in Equation 24 gives us:

$$t = \frac{165 - 100}{78.5 \sqrt{\dfrac{1}{12} + \dfrac{1}{18}}} = 2.222$$

The t statistic is dependent on sample size, so tables of t such as Appendix 7 have to be read for the appropriate number of degrees of freedom, unlike tables of z. The rule here is that, for an *unpaired* 't' test, the number of degrees of freedom is:

$$df = n_1 + n_2 - 2$$

In this example there are $(12 + 18 - 2 =)$ 28 df

From Appendix 7 we see that, for 28 df a t bigger than 2.048 is significant, $P < 0.05$. We can therefore reject the Null Hypothesis and conclude that the mean serum CKA is increased in persons taking hard regular exercise.

At first sight this calculation looks complicated, but any modern calculator with a single memory can perform the necessary steps sequentially, without the need for you to write down intermediate steps.

Paired data. If we now return to the data of Example 4.4, we can see that although the non-parametric test showed that there was a significant effect of the dietary supplement on weight, it told us nothing about the average difference, which we might want to know. It has the added disadvantage of not being an especially sensitive test. We could therefore examine the data using a *paired t-test*. This is expressed as:

$$t = \frac{\bar{x} - \mu}{s/\sqrt{n}} \qquad \text{Equation 27}$$

where $\bar{x}$ = the observed mean *difference* between the pairs

μ = the hypothetical mean difference

$s/\sqrt{n}$ = SE of the observed mean difference

The similarity with previous equations is again obvious. If there is *no* difference between the treated and untreated groups, then the *observed* mean difference, $\bar{x}$, will be approximately the same as the *expected* difference, μ, which is, of course, zero on a Null Hypothesis. We are again calculating a ratio between the amount by which the observed mean difference differs from zero and the standard error of the observed mean difference.

Example 5.4
Do the data of Example 4.4 show a statistically significant difference between the two treatment groups if a Student's 't' test is used?

H_0: There is no difference between groups

First: Calculate the mean difference. Treat the differences in Table 4.7 as x. Then:

$$\bar{x} = \frac{39.5}{9} = 4.38 \text{ g}$$

Second: Calculate the variance (s^2) and standard error of this mean difference: The short-cut way is to combine Equations 4 and 5, giving:

$$s^2 = \frac{\Sigma x^2 - [(\Sigma x)^2/n]}{n - 1} = \frac{335.25 - 173.36}{8} = 20.23$$

$$s = \sqrt{s^2} = 4.497$$

therefore,

$$SE = \frac{4.497}{\sqrt{9}} = 1.499$$

Again, even a small calculator will let you perform this calculation very easily, without writing down intermediate steps.

Third: Calculate t from Equation 27

$$t = \frac{4.38 - 0}{1.499} = 2.921$$

For a paired 't' test, use $(n - 1)$ degrees of freedom. For $(9 - 1 =) 8$ degrees of freedom, with a t of 2.921, $P < 0.02$. We therefore reject the Null Hypothesis again, but with a greater degree of confidence ($P < 0.02$ rather than $P < 0.05$).

We thus now also know what the *average* change in weight with treatment is, and its standard error (4.38 ± 1.49 g), which can be useful information.

A paired 't' test again assumes that the differences between pairs are themselves normally distributed. If, in Example 4.4, the difference in pair 9 had been 21 g, instead of 11, the Wilcoxon test would have been unaffected. In the 't' test however, the *mean* difference would have been $49.5/9 = 5.5$ g, the variance more than twice as big (47.87 compared with 20.23), and t itself would then be 2.384. This is still just significant, but to a considerably lesser degree $(P < 0.05)$ and we might begin to worry about the possibility of a Type II error (Chapter 1).

Degrees of freedom in 't' tests

There is frequently confusion over the number of degrees of freedom which should be used in 't'-tests. The general rule is that you *lose* one degree of freedom every time you calculate a variance. In a *paired* 't' test, you have calculated one variance, that of the differences between pairs, so you have:

(number of pairs minus 1) df

In an *unpaired* 't' test, you have calculated the variance of each sample so you have:

[(n_1 observations in sample 1)   + (n_2 in sample 2) minus two] df

Similarly, when using Appendix 6, you have $(n - 1)$ degrees of freedom for both numerator and denominator, since you have calculated a variance for each group.

Unpaired samples when the F test is significant

Where an F test is significant, it is not appropriate to use a normal 't' test. Instead, we revert to a z test (Equation 22). However, when we have calculated z, we look it up in the table of 't' with f degrees of freedom where:

$$f = \frac{1}{\dfrac{u^2}{n_1 - 1} + \dfrac{(1 - u)^2}{n_2 - 1}}$$

Equation 28

and

$$u = \frac{\dfrac{s^2}{n_1}}{\dfrac{s^2}{n_1} + \dfrac{s^2}{n_2}}$$

Equation 29

Although these equations look complex, in fact, they are not. Look again at Equation 28. s^2/n_1 is a kind of 'mean variance' for the measurements in the first sample, and s^2/n_2 is the same for the second sample. Equation 28 is just calculating the proportion of the sum of both 'mean variances' ($[s_1^2/n_1] + [s_2^2/n_2]$) made up by one of them. It makes no difference which group you define as Group 1 and Group 2 because Equation 27 takes both into account. Logically, u must always be less than 1, so $u + (1 - u)$ will account for both groups.

This f will be smaller than $[n_1 + n_2 - 2]$ and allows for the difference in variances. Experience will show you that it is not usually worthwhile to use this modified 'z' if the initial F test was significant $P < 0.01$. It can be useful for the grey range between $P < 0.05$ and $P < 0.01$.

Example 5.5
Imagine that the data in Example 5.3 had been as shown below

	Mean CKA	s	n
Marathon runners	175	110	12
Others	100	70	18

F is now $110^2/70^2 = 2.469$, which, from Appendix 6, is significant, $P < 0.05$. We thus use Equation 22, which gives us:

$$z = \frac{175 - 100}{\sqrt{\dfrac{110^2}{12} + \dfrac{70^2}{18}}} = 2.096$$

We now derive u from Equation 28:

$$u = \frac{\dfrac{110^2}{12}}{\dfrac{110^2}{12} + \dfrac{70^2}{18}} = 0.787$$

and substitute it in Equation 27:

$$f = \frac{1}{\dfrac{0.787^2}{11} + \dfrac{(1 - 0.787)^2}{17}} = 16.94$$

We then treat our d of 2.096 as if it were t with 17 df. Appendix 7 shows this not to be significant so, under these circumstances, we would accept the Null Hypothesis and consider that hard exercise was not statistically significantly altering serum CKA.

One- and two-tailed tests:
So far we have only been interested in testing to see whether the Null Hypothesis is tenable. We have not specified the direction in which we

expect changes to occur, and in the great majority of instances, this is the correct approach. So, in Example 4.4, the effect of the dietary supplement might have been in the other direction, being associated with smaller weights. The Null Hypothesis didn't specify 'bigger' or 'smaller', although it could have done. Usually, this non-specification is the correct approach, but occasionally it's not.

Imagine that drug D is the routine treatment for a life-threatening condition. Brown & Jones plc now produce drug E, which, they claim, gives a higher recovery rate. We are only interested in testing this claim since if it turned out to be worse, or even the same as well-tried drug D, we should not wish to change. Considered in terms of the normal distribution, instead of being interested in *both* 'tails' of the normal distribution, we are now only interested in one (Figure 5.2).

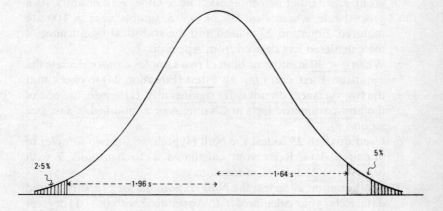

Fig. 5.2 Distribution curve showing the difference between one- and two-tailed tests of significance at the 5% level ($P < 0.05$)

Remember that $\pm 1.96s$ from the mean in *either* direction only excludes 5% of the population, i.e. 2.5% in either tail. If we are interested in looking at 5% in *one* tail, then we need to use $1.64s$, which covers 90% of the population, giving 5% in each tail. Similarly, $\pm 2.57s$ only excludes 1% of the population, 0.5% in each tail. If we are interested in looking at 1% in one tail, we would use $2.32s$.

This ensures that, in the long run, the use of one-tailed tests, where appropriate, will still mean that the modified Null Hypothesis will be rejected *when valid* only 5% or 1% or 0.5% of the time, in the instances above.

SUMMARY OF CHAPTER 5

1. This chapter deals with ways of testing departures from the Null Hypothesis for groups of data measured on an interval scale and which are approximately normally-distributed. When data is not normally-distributed, the tests described in Chapter 4 should be used.

2. When the population mean is known, and the size of the sample under investigation is greater than 30, Equation 21 can be used to test whether the sample mean differs statistically from the population mean.

3. More usually, we do not know the population mean. If we wish to assess the statistical significance of differences between the means of 2 samples, each with $n > 30$, Equation 22 is used.

4. Two percentages can be compared provided that $n > 30$ for each group and neither percentage is close to either zero or unity. As a general rule, where $P < 0.2$ or > 0.8, sample sizes > 100 are required. Equation 23 is used and the statistical significance of the calculated z is derived from Appendix 1.

5. When $n < 30$ in either or both of two samples do not calculate the z statistic. First, carry out an F test (Equation 24) to check that the two variances do not differ significantly. If they do, use one of the non-parametric tests in Chapter 4 or a modified 'z' test (see section 8).

6. Use Equation 25 to test the Null Hypothesis for two samples of unpaired data. Refer your calculated 't' to Appendix 7 with $(n_1 + n_2 - 2)$ degrees of freedom.

7. Use Equation 27 to test the Null Hypothesis for properly-paired data. Refer your calculated 't' to Appendix 7 with $(n - 1)$ degrees of freedom.

8. Use Equation 22 to test the Null Hypothesis for unpaired data where the F test is significant, $P < 0.05 > 0.01$. Do not refer your calculated 'z' to Appendix 1 but use Appendix 7 with the number of degrees of freedom calculated from Equations 28 and 29.

9. It is usual to test a Null Hypothesis with a two-tailed test, that is, excluding an equal proportion of the distribution in both 'tails' of the normal curve. Occasionally, if the only point of interest is if, for example, a treatment is a significant improvement on an alternative, then it is appropriate to use a one-tailed test, in which only the proportion of data in one 'tail' of the distribution is considered.

QUESTIONS FOR CHAPTER 5

Q1. Samples of umbilical arterial (UA) blood were obtained from 11 infants at delivery by elective Caesarean section (CS) and 36 infants at spontaneous vaginal delivery (SVD). The mean plasma noradrenaline (NOR) concentrations $\pm$ SE are summarized below. Is there a significant difference in plasma NOR concentrations depending on the method of delivery?

	Mean NOR $(nmol \cdot l^{-1})$	SE
CS	5.24	0.71
SVD	21.88	0.50

A1. H_0: The method of delivery did not significantly affect umbilical arterial concentrations of noradrenaline

We first need to back calculate from the standard errors to arrive at estimates of the variance. Rearranging Equation 8 gives:

$$s_{CS} = SE \times \sqrt{n} = 0.71 \times \sqrt{11} = 2.355$$

$$s_{SVD} = 0.50 \times \sqrt{36} = 3.00$$

The two variances are thus:

$$s_{CS}^2 = 5.55 \text{ and } s_{SVD}^2 = 9$$

$$F = \frac{9}{5.55} = 1.621 \text{ which is not significant}$$

We can therefore use Equation 25:

$$t = \frac{5.24 - 21.88}{2.869 \sqrt{\dfrac{1}{11} + \dfrac{1}{36}}} = -16.83$$

having calculated s_c from Equation 26. Appendix 7 shows that a 't' of 16.83 (ignore the sign) with 45 df is significant, $P < 0.001$. We can thus confidently reject the Null Hypothesis.

Q2. 9 infants with neonatal hyperbilirubinaemia were given ultra-violet therapy. Their serum bilirubin values $(mg \cdot dl^{-1})$ before and after therapy are summarized below. Was phototherapy associated with a change in the hyperbilirubinaemia?

Baby:	1	2	3	4	5	6	7	8	9
Before	14	15	14	16	15	14	16	14	14
After	10	12	9	14	12	9	13	11	10

A2. H_0: Phototherapy was not associated with a change in the hyperbilirubinaemia

Since the serum bilirubin concentration fell in every baby, the sign test alone (Appendix 3) shows us that a significant fall had occurred, $P < 0.05$. However, we might wish to use a test of greater sensitivity, such as a paired 't' test. We then use Equation 27, where, of course, x and s are the mean and standard deviation of the *differences* between the measurements.

$$t = \frac{3.55 - 0}{1.012/\sqrt{9}} = 10.52$$

From Appendix 7, for such a 't' with 8 df, we find $P < 0.001$ and reject the Null Hypothesis.

A word of caution about interpretation here. The perinatal period is a time of great change in the newborn. It is not safe to assume that the observed fall in serum bilirubin concentration is *due* to the phototherapy unless you also have a control group of untreated infants. This is a specific example of a general principle that needs bearing in mind.

Q3. The mean age at entry to a medical school was known to be 18.5 years. The Registrar noted one year that the mean age of the 63 students entering was 18 years 4 months, with a standard deviation of 9 months. Was this difference significant?

A3. H_0: There was no difference between the mean age at entry of the 63 students and that of previous entrants

In this instance, we treat 18.5 years as the mean age of the population (μ) of medical school entrants, and compare our sample mean with it using Equation 21, since $n > 30$. Thus:

$$z = \frac{18.33 - 18.5}{0.75/\sqrt{63}} = -1.80$$

Since this ratio is less than 1.96 (Appendix 1), we can accept the Null Hypothesis.

Q4. 273 women with anovulatory infertility were treated with one of two hormone preparations. 127 received hormone D; ovulation was successfully induced in 92. The remainder received hormone E and ovulation was induced in 118. Was there a difference in effectiveness between the two preparations?

A4. H_0: There was no difference in effectiveness

We are obviously comparing two success rates in this question, and so use Equation 23.

$$p = \frac{210}{273} = 0.769$$

'z' can therefore be calculated as:

$$z = \frac{(92/127) - (118/146)}{\sqrt{\dfrac{0.769 \times 0.231}{127} + \dfrac{0.769 \times 0.231}{146}}} = -1.638$$

We see from Appendix 1 that $z = -1.638$ is not significant; we can therefore accept the Null Hypothesis that there is no difference in ovulation induction rate in response to the two preparations.

Q5.   The mean diastolic blood pressure (BP_D) in 86 general practitioners whose body weights were above the 95th centile of weight for age was 88.6 mmHg, standard deviation 15 mmHg. The comparable figures for 90 general practitioners of a similar age range whose weights were at or below the 50th centile were 82.0, standard deviation 13 mmHg. Did the mean BP_D differ in the two groups?

A5. H_0: There was no difference in BP_D between the two groups

The number of general practitioners in both groups is greater than 30, so we use Equation 22.

$$z = \frac{88.6 - 82.0}{\sqrt{\dfrac{225}{86} + \dfrac{169}{90}}} = 3.11$$

A 'z' of 3.11 is significant, $P < 0.002$ (Appendix 1). We can therefore assume that the heavier general practitioners did have somewhat raised diastolic blood pressures.

Q6.   The results from the second year examinations of two groups of medical students, groups A and B, are shown below. Use both a non-parametric and a parametric technique to test the hypothesis that students in group A got different grades from those in group B.

Group A: 68, 82, 67, 73, 67, 60, 63, 75, 66, 78

Group B: 67, 74, 58, 59, 70, 60, 58, 54, 67, 65, 51

A6. H_0: There is no difference in grades achieved in the two groups

Non-parametric: This data is suitable for a ranking test such as Wilcoxon's ranking test for unpaired data. The results for the data as a whole are therefore *ranked* (ranks shown in bold type).

Group A: 68,   82, 67, 73, 67, 60, 63, 75, 66, 78
           15   21 12.5 17 12.5 6.5 8   19 10   20

Group B: 67,   74, 58, 59, 70, 60, 58, 54, 67, 65, 51
           12.5 18 3.5 5   16   6.5 3.5 2 12.5 9   1

$$T_1 = 141.5$$

Appendix 5 shows that when a group of $n = 10$ results, $T = 141.5$, is compared with one of $n = 11$, there is less than one chance in 20 ($P < 0.05$) of the observed distributions having come from the same population. We can thus reject the Null Hypothesis.

Parametric: An unpaired 't' test should be suitable here. The variance for Group A can be calculated to be 47.65, while that for Group B is 49.69. Therefore:

$$F = \frac{49.69}{47.65} = 1.04$$

which is not significant, confirming the suitability of a 't' test.

$$s_c^2 = \frac{(47.65 \times 9) + (49.69 \times 10)}{10 + 11 - 2} = 48.72$$

$$s_c = \sqrt{48.72} = 6.979$$

't' is now calculated from Equation 25:

$$t = \frac{69.9 - 62.1}{6.979 \sqrt{\dfrac{1}{10} + \dfrac{1}{11}}} = 2.557$$

We have ($10 + 11 - 2 =$) 19 df and see that, from Appendix 7, $P < 0.02$. We can thus reject the Null Hypothesis.

Q7. A group of 20 poorly-controlled diabetic patients were found to have a mean fasting blood glucose (FBG) concentration of $8.7 \, \text{mmol} \cdot l^{-1}$, standard deviation $1.8 \, \text{mmol} \cdot l^{-1}$. The FBG in 20 non-diabetic patients was $3.7 \, \text{mmol} \cdot l^{-1}$, standard deviation $1.1 \, \text{mmol} \cdot l^{-1}$. Calculate the degree of significance for the difference between these two samples.

A7. H_0: There is no difference between the two mean FBG concentrations

$$F = \frac{1.8^2}{1.1^2} = 2.678$$

Appendix 6 shows this to be significant, $P < 0.05$. We thus use the 'z' statistic (Equation 22), but refer it to Appendix 7 with f degrees of freedom, derived from Equations 28 and 29.

$$z = \frac{8.7 - 3.7}{\sqrt{\dfrac{1.8^2}{20} + \dfrac{1.1^2}{20}}} = 10.59$$

$$u = \frac{1.8^2/20}{1.8^2/20 + 1.1^2/20} = 0.728$$

$$f = \frac{1}{\dfrac{0.728^2}{19} + \dfrac{(1 - 0.728)^2}{19}} = 31.46$$

Appendix 7 shows a 't' (z in this instance) of 10.59 with 31 df to be highly statistically significant, $P < 0.001$.

Q8. A hospital laboratory quoted a normal mean value for serum vitamin B_{12} concentration of $350 \, \text{pg} \cdot ml^{-1}$. Mean serum B_{12} measured in 45 strict vegetarians was $290 \, \text{pg} \cdot ml^{-1}$ with a standard deviation of $90 \, \text{pg} \cdot ml^{-1}$. Is the mean serum B_{12} concentration significantly altered in vegetarians?

A8. H_0: There is no difference between the sample and population means

Using Equation 21, we calculate:

$$z = \frac{290 - 350}{90/\sqrt{45}} = -4.47$$

We see from Appendix 1 that there is less than one chance in

5 000 ($P < 0.0005$) of a sample of 45 patients having a mean serum B_{12} concentration of 290 and a standard deviation of 90 pg $\cdot$ ml^{-1} having come from the 'normal' population. We thus reject the Null Hypothesis. However, since the mean value of 290 pg $\cdot$ ml^{-1} is considerably higher than the lower end of the normal range (150 pg $\cdot$ ml^{-1}) the *clinical* significance of the result is likely to be small, even though the *statistical* significance is high.

Q9. The mean total albumin concentration at term of the 32 women in Example 5.2 is shown below. What was the effect of a previous pregnancy on mean total albumin concentration?

1st pregnancy: mean 3.1 g $\cdot$ dl^{-1}, s 0.38

2nd pregnancy: mean 2.9 g $\cdot$ dl^{-1}, s 0.45

A9. H_0: Parity did not influence mean total albumin concentration

The numbers of patients in each sample are greater than 30 so we can use Equation 22.

$$z = \frac{3.1 - 2.9}{\sqrt{\dfrac{0.38^2}{32} + \dfrac{0.45^2}{32}}} = 1.920$$

We see from Appendix 1 that a z of 1.92 is not statistically significant, $P > 0.05$. We thus accept the Null Hypothesis.

6

A brief introduction to the analysis of variance

In our original discussion of the normal distribution (Chapter 2), we saw that the sample mean, $\bar{x}$, and standard deviation, s, which we calculate, are used as approximations for the hypothetical population mean, μ, and standard deviation, σ. In Chapter 5 we saw that if two sample means differed by more than a certain amount in relation to a 'combined standard error' then we could conclude that they had not been drawn from the same population. These tests require the assumption that the sample variances are not significantly different, and it is to test this that we use the F test (Equation 24).

If the F test is significant, then we again have to assume that there is something different about the populations from which our samples have been drawn. This very simple test of equality of variance can be expanded to allow the comparison of several samples with each other, not only in terms of their variance, but also in terms of their mean values.

Experiments such as those in the evaluation of a new drug are comparing the effect of different treatments on different groups. Basic analysis of variance allows a quick comparison of several groups at once. There are two distinct sources of variability, the natural variability *within* each group, and the variability *between* groups caused by treatment. The analysis of variance is simply used to decide whether the observed overall variation can be accounted for merely by within group variation, or whether some must have arisen as a result of the treatment. This is most easily discussed in terms of an example.

Example 6.1
18 consecutive pregnant patients with diastolic blood pressures between 90 and 100 mmHg at 30 weeks gestation were allocated *either* to treatment with bed-rest alone, (Group A) *or* to treatment with bed-rest and drug X (Group B) *or* to treatment with bed-rest and drug Y (Group C). The *fall* in diastolic blood pressure (x) after 3 days of treatment is summarized below.

| | Group A (n = 6) | | Group B (n = 6) | | Group C (n = 6) | |
	x	x^2	x	x^2	x	x^2
	6	36	10	100	13	169
	4	16	11	121	14	196
	5	25	9	81	11	121
	3	9	11	121	10	100
	4	16	12	144	12	144
	4	16	13	169	13	169
Group totals:	26	118	66	736	73	899
Means:	4.33		11.0		12.17	

Overall totals: $\Sigma x_{A,B,C} = 165$

$\Sigma x^2_{A,B,C} = 1753$

Before we can calculate the 'within group' and 'between group' variances, we need to calculate their sums of squares ($\Sigma(x - \bar{x})^2$; Chapter 2 and Equation 5). This is most easily done by *first* calculating the *total* sum of squares and then that *between treatments*. Subtracting the second from the first then gives us the 'within group' or 'residual' sum of squares. The *total* sum of squares is:

$$\Sigma(x - \bar{x})^2 = \Sigma x^2_{A,B,C} - \frac{(\Sigma x_{A,B,C})^2}{n_{A,B,C}} = 1753 - \frac{165^2}{18} = 240.5$$

The sum of squares *between treatments* is calculated from:

$$\frac{(\Sigma x_A)^2}{n_A} + \frac{(\Sigma x_B)^2}{n_B} + \frac{(\Sigma x_C)^2}{n_C} - \frac{(\Sigma x_{A,B,C})^2}{n_{A,B,C}}$$

Be very careful about what you are squaring. $(\Sigma x_A)^2$ means (26 × 26 =) 676 which is *not* the same as Σx^2_A which is 118. Thus:

$\Sigma(x - \bar{x})^2$ between treatments

$$= \frac{26^2}{6} + \frac{66^2}{6} + \frac{73^2}{6} - \frac{165^2}{18}$$

$$= 214.3$$

The next stage is to set out an *analysis of variance table* as shown in Table 6.1.

We have calculated the total sum of squares and the between treatment sum of squares; the residual is then calculated by simple subtraction. The *total* number of degrees of freedom are $(n - 1)$ because we calculated a single total variance. We also calculated

Table 6.1 Analysis of variance table for the data of Example 6.1

Source of variation	Sum of squares	Degrees of freedom	Mean square (variance)	Variance ratio (F)
Between treatments	214.3	2	107.15	61.33
Residual (within group)	26.2	15	1.747	
Total	240.5	17		

individual variances for each of the treatments; the number of degrees of freedom here is thus $(m - 1)$ where m is the number of treatment groups, 3 in this example. The difference between these two degrees of freedom then gives us the residual degrees of freedom. We can then calculate the variances as usual from:

$$s^2 = \frac{\Sigma(x - \bar{x})^2}{\mathrm{df}}$$ Equation 4

and calculate the ratio between the variances arising from the two sources of variation. We then use Appendix 6 with $f_1 = 2$ and $f_2 = 15$, and see that an F of 61.33 means that there is much less than one chance in 100 ($P < 0.01$) of all of the samples having come from the same population.

Note that all that this tells us is that there *are* differences between the treatment groups, not where the differences lie, nor whether each treatment is different from every other. If we wish to compare, say, Groups A and C, we simply use Equation 25. Under these circumstances, s is the square root of the *residual* variance. Thus:

$$t = \frac{\dfrac{26}{6} - \dfrac{73}{6}}{\sqrt{1.747}\sqrt{\dfrac{1}{6} + \dfrac{1}{6}}} = \frac{4.33 - 12.17}{1.321\sqrt{0.33}} = -10.33$$

Under these circumstances you use $(n_T - m)$ degrees of freedom, i.e. 15.

The necessary calculations for an analysis of variance of m treatments each having n observations (n need not be the same in each group) of some response variable, x, can be summarized as below, where:

n_T = total number of observations

$n_1, n_2, ..., n_m$ = number in individual treatment groups

Σx_T = total of all xs

$\Sigma x_1, \Sigma x_2, ..., \Sigma x_m$ = total of the xs in each treatment group

The total sum of squares about the mean is given by:

$$\Sigma x_T^2 - \frac{(\Sigma x_T)^2}{n_T} \qquad \text{Equation 5}$$

The 'between treatment' sum of squares is given by:

$$\frac{(\Sigma x_1)^2}{n_1} + \frac{(\Sigma x_2)^2}{n_2} + ... + \frac{(\Sigma x_m)^2}{n_m} - \frac{(\Sigma x_T)^2}{n_T} \qquad \text{Equation 30}$$

As you can see, the basic calculations needed are not difficult provided you keep a clear head! It is almost invariably helpful to set out the individual data as in Example 6.1, so that the various totals can be clearly identified and to remember that small calculators will accumulate both Σx and Σx^2.

Much more could be said about the analysis of variance, but it would not be appropriate in a book of this kind. It is often possible to design experiments which can utilise the analysis of variance to test hypotheses. This is an area in which, once again, expert statistical help in relation to your specific question is invaluable. Such help is one of the *raisons d'être* for University statisticians. Make the most of it!

SUMMARY OF CHAPTER 6

1. The analysis of variance is used to establish whether the observed amount of variation between treatment groups is greater than would be expected to occur if all samples had been drawn from the same population, that is, if treatment was without effect on the measured variable.
2. This is achieved by the separate calculation of the total sums of squares and the 'between group' sums of squares, using Equations 5 and 30. The 'within group' sum of squares is then obtained by subtraction.
3. The 'between group' and 'within group' variances are then calculated as usual from Equation 4, and the ratio between them (F) determined. This is then referred to Appendix 6.
4. The mean values of the measured variable in any two treatment groups can then be tested for departure from the Null Hypothesis using Equation 25.

QUESTIONS FOR CHAPTER 6

Q1. A medical student obtained the following data concerning birthweight at term and maternal smoking habits. Use an analysis of variance to determine whether, from these data, smoking influences birthweight.

Smoking habit (cigarettes/day)	0	1–15	16–39	≥ 40
Body weight (kg):	3.5	3.0	2.8	2.5
	3.2	2.9	2.9	2.6
	2.8	3.1	2.7	2.2
	3.0	2.8	3.0	2.3
	2.9	3.0	2.5	2.4
	3.1	3.2	2.7	
	3.4	3.1		

A1. H_0: Bodyweight was not affected by smoking habit

First calculate n_T, Σx_T, Σx and Σx^2 for each smoking group. Then:

$$\Sigma(x - \bar{x})^2_T = 207.6 - \frac{(71.6)^2}{25} = 2.538$$

and $\Sigma(x - \bar{x})^2$ between groups

$$= \frac{(21.9)^2}{7} + \ldots + \frac{(12)^2}{5} - \frac{(71.6)^2}{25} = 1.781$$

Construct a table for the analysis of variance. From this it will be seen that the 'between group' variance is $(1.781/3 =) 0.593$, while the 'residual' variance is $(0.757/21 =) 0.0360$. The variance ratio, F, is thus:

$$F = \frac{0.593}{0.036} = 16.47$$

Reject the Null Hypothesis, $P \ll 0.01$.

Q2. Using the data in Q1, test whether the mean birthweight differs:

a) between non-smoking mothers and those smoking up to 15 cigarettes per day
b) between non-smoking mothers and those smoking more than 40 cigarettes per day

A2. The Null Hypothesis is the same in both instances, that is:

H_0: Smoking is not associated with a change in birthweight

Substituting in Equation 25 gives:

a)
$$t = \frac{3.129 - 3.014}{0.19 \sqrt{\dfrac{1}{7} + \dfrac{1}{7}}} = 1.133$$

This is not significant, with 21 df. $(P > 0.1)$—accept the Null Hypothesis

b)
$$t = \frac{3.129 - 2.40}{0.19 \sqrt{\dfrac{1}{7} + \dfrac{1}{5}}} = 6.552$$

This, however, is significant, $P < 0.001$—reject the Null Hypothesis.

7

Correlation and regression

Up to now we have been interested mainly in descriptive and comparative statistics. The last major type we shall consider here are those allowing us to assess the degree of *association* or *correlation* between two variables. A common use is for testing for any relationship between the administered dose of a substance, and the evoked response. Under these circumstances we have effectively set up an experiment in which by altering one variable we expect to change another, that is, we are testing for *cause and effect*. The other circumstances in which indices of association are frequently used is when data have been collected from non-experimental situations, and there are theoretical grounds for thinking that there may be an association between variables. Measurements of height and weight or smoking habits and blood pressure are examples of this second type.

A word of warning. This chapter tells you how to test for a *statistically* significant correlation between two variables. *The existence of a statistically significant correlation cannot be taken as evidence of causality* in relation to non-experimental data. All it can do is to indicate a possibility which, if it is of potential value, may be worth testing experimentally. For example, suppose that you had collected data on the number of bronchitic attacks suffered in a winter in a large group of patients. You might find a range of number of attacks which showed a general association with smoking habit. You are not surprised. What does surprise you is that there also appears to be an association between the number of mints eaten per day and the number of bronchitic attacks. What you have failed to realise is that there is a flourishing 'Smokers Anonymous' in the town, and that many of the mint-eaters are trying to wean themselves off tobacco. You are looking at the residual effects of a quite different stimulus.

χ^2 yet again
We saw in Chapters 3 and 4 that the χ^2 statistic lets us test whether the *observed* number of occurrences in any cell of a contingency table such as Table 4.2 differs significantly from those which would be

expected on the Null Hypothesis. This is, in a way, looking for an association between the variable in the columns and the variable in the rows, and can be useful, especially when dealing with nominal data. A brief example will remind you of the technique.

Example 7.1

It is a matter of common observation that there is a degree of association between hair colour and eye colour. Do the data from a random sample of 400 students displayed in Table 7.1 lend statistically significant support to this observation?

The expected number in each cell has been calculated as described in Chapter 3. So, for example, 240 students have brown hair and 40 have hazel eyes. We would thus expect:

$$\frac{240 \times 40}{400} = 24 \text{ students}$$

to have the colouring 'brown hair/hazel eyes' if there were no association between the two variables, which is, of course, our Null Hypothesis.

We then simply calculate χ^2 from Equation 11 as usual.

Table 7.1 Data concerning hair and eye colour in a sample of 400 students. The 'expected' values are shown in bold type.

Hair colour Eye colour	Fair	Brown	Black	Totals
Blue	80 **50**	116 **120**	4 **30**	200
Hazel	16 **10**	18 **24**	6 **6**	40
Brown	4 **40**	106 **96**	50 **24**	160
Totals	100	240	60	400

$$\chi^2 = \frac{(80 - 50)^2}{50} + \frac{(116 - 120)^2}{120} + \dots + \frac{(50 - 24)^2}{24}$$

$$= 107.4$$

This has $(3 - 1) \times (3 - 1)\,\text{df} = 4$ degrees of freedom

From Appendix 2 we see that a value greater than 18.5 will only occur on average in less than 1 in 1000 samples. We can therefore confidently say that there is an association between hair colour and eye colour in the sample considered, and reject the Null Hypothesis.

Spearman's rank correlation coefficient

It frequently happens that when we have two sets of interval data, for example, gestation length and urinary oestriol concentration, one of these sets is not normally distributed. This occurs especially often with hormone measurements. In this instance, we can *either* try to normalise the skewed distribution using, for example log_{10}, *or* we can use a ranking method to assess whether the two are in some way associated.   NON - PARAMETRIC

Example 7.2

The ages and weights at booking for 10 primigravidae are shown in Table 7.2. Is there a significant association between weight and age?

Table 7.2 Ages and weights at booking of 10 primigravidae

Patient	R_a	Age	Weight	R_w	$(R_a - R_w) = D$	D^2
Q	1	17	43	1	0	0
M	2	19	59	5	−3	9
N	3	20	57	4	−1	1
P	4.5	21	55	3	+1.5	2.25
K	4.5	21	68	10	−5.5	30.25
L	6.5	22	60	6	+0.5	0.25
S	6.5	22	61	7	−0.5	0.25
F	8	23	54	2	+6	36
D	9	24	63	8	+1	1
A	10	25	64	9	+1	1
Totals						81

H_0: Basal body weight is not influenced by age

If this hypothesis were valid, then the *ranks* for weight (R_w) would be entirely randomly distributed, and would in no way run parallel with the ranks for age (R_a). Conversely, if age completely determined weight, the ranks for age and weight would be identical. *Spearman's ρ* [pronounced 'roh'] which is also known as r_S, gives a measure of how well the ranks agree (their *concordance*).

First, note the rank order for each measurement, starting with the smallest. Then calculate the difference between R_a and R_w for each patient. This is then a new variable called D (difference). Because some Ds are negative and some positive, they are then squared. The sum of the D^2 (ΣD^2) is then calculated.

Spearman's ρ is given by:

$$\rho = 1 - \frac{(6 \times \Sigma D^2)}{n(n^2 - 1)} \qquad \text{Equation 31}$$

Substituting in Equation 31:

$$\rho = \frac{6 \cdot \times 81}{10 \times (10^2 - 1)} = \frac{486}{990} = 0.4909$$

If the ranks agreed absolutely, every D would be 0, so every D^2 would be 0 and ρ would be $+1$. Conversely, you may like to work out for yourself that if there were complete *negative concordance*, with the youngest patient being the heaviest and so on through to the oldest being the lightest, ρ would be -1. Do remember that the phrase 'a negative correlation' does not mean 'no statistically significant correlation' but rather, that one variable increases as the other decreases (Fig. 7.1). A random distribution will result in values of ρ close to 0. Appendix 8 shows the values of ρ required to establish a

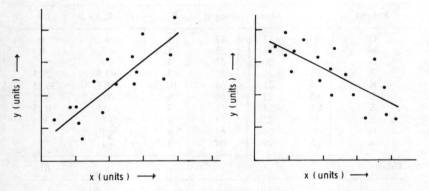

Fig. 7.1 Two scattergrams of data measured on interval scales, illustrating that an association between variables can be either positive (left hand side) or negative (inverse; right hand side). The lines of best fit have been drawn in by eye.

significant departure from the Null Hypothesis for up to 30 pairs. Note that in Appendix 8, n is the actual number of pairs under study. In Example 7.2, the observed ρ of 0.4909 will occur by chance more than 1 in 10 times, so we would accept the Null Hypothesis.

When the sample is bigger than 30, tables of r (Appendix 9; see below) are used.

Correlation
We come finally to the assessment of degrees of association between two variables measured on interval scales, *both having normal distributions.* This last phrase is most important; if one or both of the variables is not normally-distributed, then it should either be transformed (Chapter 2) or Spearman's ρ, a non-parametric test of

association, should be used. Regression analysis (see below) can also be used sometimes for data where a variable is not normally-distributed.

Logically-speaking, variables such as age, time, gestation length, drug dose etc are *independent* variables. A baby's bodyweight will increase with age, but his age is unaffected by changes in bodyweight. These independent variables are plotted on the horizontal or x axis of a scattergram and are thus known as x variables. The *dependent* variables, those which may be proportional to the independent variables, are plotted on the vertical or y axis, and are known as y variables. It is a good practice to plot out your raw data as in Figure 7.2 before beginning any analysis. This allows you visually to assess whether there may indeed be an association between the variables, and if so, whether it is in the form of a straight line or curved. It also lets you check that both variables are roughly normally distributed.

For any sample consisting of n pairs of data, an independent, x, and a dependent, y, variable, we need to calculate the mean and sums of squares for each variable ($\bar{x}$, $\Sigma(x - \bar{x})^2$ and $\bar{y}$, $\Sigma(y - \bar{y})^2$). This gives us

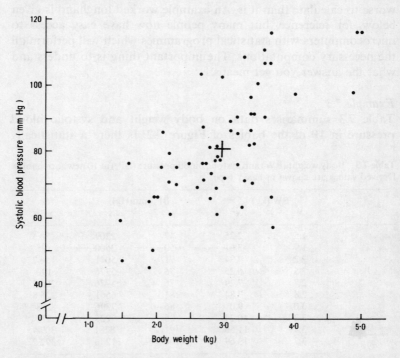

Fig. 7.2 Scattergram of data concerning body weight at birth (x axis) and systolic blood pressure (y axis) in 60 newborn infants

our ordinary measure of central tendency of the data. The mean values are marked as + on Figure 7.2. We also need to calculate the sum of the products of each x and y, Σxy and the sum of the products about the means, $\Sigma(x - \bar{x})(y - \bar{y})$.

We can calculate $\Sigma(x - \bar{x})^2$ and $\Sigma(y - \bar{y})^2$ from Equation 5 as usual. $\Sigma(x - \bar{x})(y - \bar{y})$ is calculated in exactly the same format, using:

$$\Sigma(x - \bar{x})(y - \bar{y}) = \Sigma xy - \frac{(\Sigma x)(\Sigma y)}{n} \qquad \text{Equation 32}$$

If $\Sigma(x - \bar{x})(y - \bar{y})$ were to be divided by $n - 1$, we would get a kind of 'product variance' known as the *covariance*. The similarity with Equation 4 is obvious.

The correlation coefficient, r, is then calculated as:

$$r = \frac{\Sigma(x - \bar{x})(y - \bar{y})}{\sqrt{\Sigma(x - \bar{x})^2 \, \Sigma(y - \bar{y})^2}} \qquad \text{Equation 33}$$

As with so many basic statistical calculations, this looks much worse to calculate than it is. An example worked longhand is given below, for reference, but many people now have easy access to microcomputers with statistical programmes which will perform all the necessary computations. The important thing is to understand what the answer you get means.

Example 7.3
Table 7.3 summarises data on body weight and systolic blood pressure in 10 of the babies of Figure 7.2. Is there a statistically

Table 7.3 Body weight (BW) and systolic blood pressure (BP_s) in 10 newborn babies. Derived values are shown in heavy type.

	BW (kg)		BP_s (mmHg)		
	x	x^2	y	y^2	$x \cdot y$
	1.5	2.25	47	2209	70.5
	1.9	3.61	50	2500	95
	2.2	4.84	71	5041	156.2
	2.5	6.25	76	5776	190
	2.7	7.29	76	5776	205.2
	2.8	7.84	81	6561	226.8
	3.0	9.0	86	7396	258
	3.2	10.24	85	7225	272
	3.4	11.56	91	8281	309.4
	3.7	13.69	106	11236	392.2
Totals:	**26.9**	**76.57**	**769**	**62001**	**2175.3**

significant association between these two variables?

The various sums of squares are calculated from Equations 5 and 32. Thus:

$$\Sigma(x - \bar{x})^2 = 76.57 - \frac{26.9^2}{10} = 4.209$$

$$\Sigma(y - \bar{y})^2 = 62001 - \frac{769^2}{10} = 2864.9$$

$$\Sigma(x - \bar{x})(y - \bar{y}) = 2175.3 - \frac{26.9 \times 769}{10} = 106.69$$

Substituting in Equation 33 gives us:

$$r = \frac{106.69}{\sqrt{4.209 \times 2864.9}} = 0.9716$$

This correlation coefficient is very close to 1. From Appendix 9 we see that an r of 0.9716 with $(n - 2)$ degrees of freedom (because we have two variances) will arise by chance in less than 1 in 1000 times ($P < 0.001$) if the Null Hypothesis is valid. We can thus say that there is a statistically significant correlation between the two variables.

A useful point to remember is that if we square r, this gives us a measure of the variation of y which can be attributed to its relationship with x. Thus, if r were $+ 1.0$, so r^2 would be 1 (which is the same as 100%) which means that all the variation of y could be accounted for in terms of x. If r were to equal $+0.7071$, r^2 would be 0.5 or 50%. Thus half the variation of y could be accounted for in terms of x, but other factors would also be important. If r were to be $- 0.4472$, r^2 would be 0.2 or 20%. In this instance, although there could still be a significant degree of correlation between x and y, 80% of the variation would not be related to changes in x.

In Example 7.3, we considered only the effect of one variable, bodyweight, on systolic blood pressure. We might however want to consider the effect of another variable, such as gestation age, as well. Bodyweight at birth will itself be partly determined by gestation age, so that we have a group of inter-related variables. The association between any two of these variables, allowing for the effect of one or more others, can be investigated using partial correlation analysis. This is beyond the scope of this introduction, but is clearly described in *Statistical Methods in Biology* by N. T. J. Bailey (see *Suggested Further Reading*).

Linear regression analysis

The question: 'Is there a statistically-significant association between these two variables?' automatically runs on to: 'If there is, by how much does a change in one variable evoke a change in the other?'. *Regression analysis* allows us to answer the second of these questions.

In carrying out regression analysis, the assumption of a normal distribution for the independent variable may not be valid. We may for example have decided to examine the response of our dependent variable to graded doses of x in 10 patients. We will then have 10 values of y for each x (dose). Regression analysis assumes a normal distribution for y, but accepts that x may have been determined on by the investigator and need not be normally distributed.

From this data, we calculate a mean y ($\bar{y}$) for each (fixed) x, and can then determine by how much *on average* y will increase for a unit rise in x. Figure 7.3 summarizes the constants which are calculated when it is assumed that the association between y and x follows a straight line. This is the most easily-handled situation, and the determination of the constants a and b is known as *linear* regression analysis. If, on looking at your raw data, plotted as a scattergram, it appears that any relationship may follow a curve, try the effect of changing the scale for

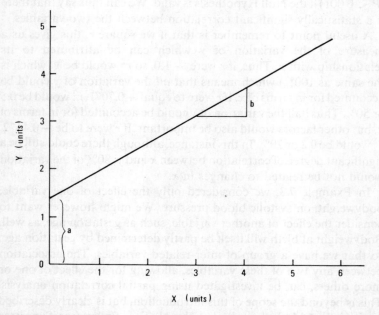

Fig. 7.3 Illustration of the values of the constants a and b in the equation for linear regression: $y = a + bx$

one of the variables. Again, $\log_{10}$ is a very useful transformation, as is the square or the square root of one of the variables. If such a replot 'straightens' the picture, then substitute $\log_{10} x$ or $1/y$ or whatever for the appropriate variable in your calculations.

The gradient, b, and the intercept on the y axis at $x = 0$, a, are calculated from:

$$b = \frac{\Sigma(x - \bar{x})(y - \bar{y})}{\Sigma(x - \bar{x})^2} \qquad \text{Equation 34}$$

and

$$a = \bar{y} - b\bar{x} \qquad \text{Equation 35}$$

These values are then substituted in the equation:

$$y = a + bx \qquad \text{Equation 36}$$

which allows us to draw the 'line of best fit' (regression line) on our scattergram.

The quantity, $\Sigma(x - \bar{x})(y - \bar{y})$ is calculated exactly as in Equation 32, and $\Sigma(x - \bar{x})^2$ as in Equation 5.

To illustrate this, consider again the data in Example 7.3. The gradient of the calculated line relating systolic blood pressure to bodyweight is given by:

$$b = \frac{106.69}{4.209} = 25.35$$

This tells us that a one kilogram increase in birth weight is associated with an average increase in systolic blood pressure of 25.35 mmHg. This is known as the regression of systolic blood pressure on birthweight. The intercept, a, is given by:

$$a = 76.9 - (25.35 \times 2.69) = 8.71$$

It would, of course, also be *theoretically* possible to calculate the average change in x for a unit change in y. When x is, as frequently, an *independent* variable, this would be a logical absurdity, but there are circumstances when it can be useful. In this case, we would calculate:

$$b = \frac{\Sigma(x - \bar{x})(y - \bar{y})}{\Sigma(y - \bar{y})^2}$$

which is then the *regression* of x on y. The two possible regressions will be identical only when $r = 1.0$. In all other instances the slopes will differ depending on the scatter of xs and ys.

We are now in a position to calculate what the average systolic blood pressure would be at any birth weight, using Equation 36. So, for example, with a birth weight of 3.5 kg, the calculated systolic blood pressure will be:

$$y = 8.71 + (25.35 \times 3.5) = 97.44 \, \text{mmHg}$$

By choosing 3 values of x within our data range, we can superimpose the 'line of best fit' on our data, as shown in Figure 7.4.

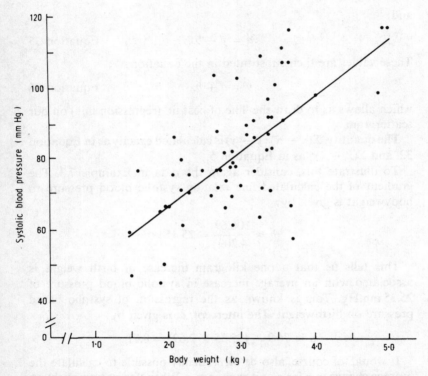

Fig. 7.4 Data as in Figure 7.2, with the superimposed line of best fit derived from: Systolic blood pressure = 35.9 + (15.0 × bodyweight). In this example, the correlation coefficient, r_c, is 0.6865, $P < 0.001$

We should also be able to quote a standard deviation about our regression line. Assuming that the variances of the ys for any given x do not change significantly from one x to another, the *variance* about the line is given by:

$$s_r^2 = \frac{1}{n-2} \left\{ \Sigma(y - y)^2 - \frac{[\Sigma(x - \bar{x})(y - \bar{y})]^2}{\Sigma(x - x)^2} \right\} \quad \text{Equation 37}$$

The standard deviation, s_r, is then of course $\sqrt{s_r^2}$. Note that this is the same for any calculated y over the entire spread of the data.

Incidentally, the assumption that the variance of the distribution of y for any given x does not change over the range of x is frequently invalid, especially when y is a biochemical variable, such as a hormone concentration. To be on the safe side, you should, as previously said, always plot your data out as a scattergram and *look* at it, before feeding it into a computer. The computer will always give you an answer, but it may be meaningless!

When n is greater than 30, the standard error of b is given by:

$$SE_b = \frac{s_r}{\sqrt{\Sigma(x - \bar{x})^2}} \qquad \text{Equation 38}$$

using the estimate of standard deviation derived from Equation 37

Significance of b. When we want to see whether our calculated b is significantly different from zero, we can test it in the same way as we assess whether the mean of a sample differs significantly from the population mean. In the case of b, the population mean on the Null Hypothesis is zero (no association). The specific test required then depends on your sample size. If n is less than 30, then we calculate t from:

$$t = \frac{b - 0}{s/\sqrt{\Sigma(x - \bar{x})^2}} \qquad \text{Equation 39}$$

Thus, in Example 7.3,

$$t = \frac{25.35 - 0}{4.4793 \sqrt{4.209}} = 2.7585$$

which, with 8 degrees of freedom we see from Appendix 7 to be significant, $P < 0.05$. Because fewer assumptions of normality are made for regression analysis, it is a less sensitive test of association than the calculation of correlation coefficients, but it is frequently more appropriate.

When n is greater than 30, tables of z (Appendix 1) can be used to determine whether the ratio calculated from Equation 39 indicates a significant departure from the Null Hypothesis.

Extrapolation
One last point. When you are drawing a regression line *do not* extrapolate the line beyond your data points. You have no evidence of what happens beyond your data so it is quite unjustifiable to extrapolate. In the first year of life, an infant roughly trebles its birth

weight. Were you to extrapolate data concerning weight and age over this period to the third birthday, you would conclude that the average 2-year-old child would weigh 30, and the 3-year-old child, 90 kg. They don't!

SUMMARY OF CHAPTER 7

1. The calculation of the various coefficients of association allows us to assess the degree of association between two normally-distributed variables. However, statistically significant coefficients are, at most, merely pointers to a possible 'cause and effect' and should not be treated as anything else.

2. The χ^2 statistic (Equation 11) allows assessment of the degree of association between variables which are not normally distributed, or between those measured on nominal or ordinal scales.

3. Spearman's rank correlation coefficient, ρ (Equation 31) is also suitable for use with non-parametric data, or variables which are not normally distributed. Appendix 8 shows the values of ρ required to establish a significant departure from the Null Hypothesis.

4. Any coefficient of association can range between -1 and $+1$. The closer it is to either end of the range, the greater the degree of association. Conversely, a value close to 0 indicates no association. When negative values are encountered, the association is said to be 'inverse', or, 'negative'. The phrase 'a negative correlation' does not mean 'no statistically significant correlation' but rather that one variable increases as the other decreases.

5. The calculation of correlation coefficients for data measured on an interval scale should properly only be performed on samples in which both variables under study are normally-distributed. It is usual to regard the independent variable as giving the x axis on a scattergram, with the dependent variable on the y axis.

6. The correlation coefficient, r, is calculated from Equation 33, with $(n-2)$ degrees of freedom. Appendix 9 shows the values of r required to establish a significant departure from the Null Hypothesis. The value r^2 gives a measure of the proportion of the total variation in y resulting from variation in x.

7. Regression analysis allows the calculation of the slope (b) of the line relating y to x (Equation 34) and the intercept on the y axis (a) (Equation 35). These two parameters allow the calculation of a line of best fit for the data, using Equation 36. It is not a prime

requirement that x shall have a normal distribution for a regression analysis.

8. The variance about the regression line is given by Equation 37. The standard error of the regression coefficient, b, is derived from Equation 38. A slightly modified 't' test (Equation 39) is used to determine whether the slope of the regression line differs significantly from zero, i.e., whether there is evidence for an association between the two variables.

9. Do not extrapolate a calculated regression line beyond your data points. You don't have any evidence of what happens to the association beyond them.

QUESTIONS FOR CHAPTER 7

Q1. Shown below are data relating to simultaneous measurements of diastolic blood pressure and heart rate in response to the infusion of a pressor hormone. Use a non-parametric test to determine whether these two variables are statistically-significantly correlated.

BP_D mmHg	84	81	87	94	70	90	76	86
HR bpm	53	63	50	48	77	56	71	63

A1. H_0: There is no association between diastolic blood pressure (BP_D) and heart rate (HR)

Spearman's ρ could be calculated here. First, rank the variables.

BP_D	R_B	HR	R_H	D	D^2
70	1	77	8	−7	49
76	2	71	7	−5	25
81	3	63	5.5	−2.5	6.25
84	4	53	3	1	1
86	5	63	5.5	−0.5	0.25
87	6	50	2	4	16
90	7	56	4	3	9
94	8	48	1	7	49

Spearman's ρ is calculated from Equation 31 as:

$$\rho = 1 - \frac{6 \times 155.5}{8 \times 63} = -0.8511$$

Appendix 8 shows that this ρ is significant for 8 data pairs, $P < 0.02$. We should thus reject the Null Hypothesis.

Q2. The calculated slope of the line relating systolic blood pressure to the body weight in 60 infants was $12.7 \text{ mmHg} \cdot \text{kg}^{-1}$ with a standard error of 2.4. Is there evidence for a significant departure from the Null Hypothesis?

A2. H_0: There is no association between systolic blood pressure and the body weight

Use Equation 39 to test H_0. Then:

$$t = \frac{12.7 - 0}{2.4} = 5.29$$

Since $n = 60$, we can use Appendix 1, and see that such a ratio would arise much less than 1 in 1000 times if the Null Hypothesis were tenable. We therefore reject the Null Hypothesis.

Q3. The regression line for the data relating systolic blood pressure to body weight in the 60 infants of Q2, had the calculated parameters:

Intercept on the y axis $(a) = 47.3$
Slope $(b) = 12.7$

What will be the average systolic blood pressure of infants weighing 2.5 and 4.0 kg?

A3. Use Equation 36. The systolic blood pressure (y) in the baby of 2.5 kg is given by:

$$y = 47.3 + (12.7 \times 2.5) = 79.1 \text{ mmHg}$$

and in the baby of 4.0 kg:

$$y = 47.3 + (12.7 \times 4.0) = 98.1 \text{ mmHg}$$

Q4. What proportion of the variation in red cell mass per kilogram bodyweight could be accounted for by its association with the haematocrit $(r = 0.768)$?

A4. $r^2 = 0.59$ so 59% of the variation in red cell mass per kilogram could occur in relation to the haematocrit.

8

Pitfalls for the unwary

This last, brief, chapter is not concerned with statistical techniques. It is a reminder of a few of the common sense concepts which are, all too often, forgotten in the rush to acquire and analyse data.

1. Inappropriate design or sampling techniques
The importance of experimental design and of the sampling techniques used cannot be overemphasised. A well-designed study will require substantially less effort to arrive at a conclusion than a poorly designed one, which may indeed be incapable of answering your question. So, first of all, formalise the question you are asking and draw up a protocol of the way in which you think you could set about answering it. The next thing to do is to discuss it with either a statistician, or someone familiar with this kind of problem. *Do not* leave this step until you have collected your data.

2. Control groups
This, of course, runs straight on from (1). Are you going to be able to collect properly paired data, or are you simply going to have to match your control group as carefully as possible to your experimental groups? Define the factors which you are going to match, and stick to them.

What about cross-over, blind and double-blind trials? These can be extremely useful in comparing treatment regimes, or comparing placebo with treatment.

3. Choice of statistical techniques
This is determined, to a considerable extent, by your data, and again, expert advice is invaluable. You should have an idea of how big your study groups are going to be; if you are looking for very small differences, your sample size will obviously need to be bigger than if the expected difference is large. If you are contemplating using χ^2, remember that your smallest *expected* number should not be less than

5, and that you must work in actual figures, not rates or percentages.

Normally-distributed data is preferably examined in terms of the standard normal deviate, z. This means that your sample sizes should be greater than 30 where possible. Smaller samples can be considered in terms of the 't' distribution, but the possibility of Type II error (wrongly accepting the Null Hypothesis) increases sharply as sample size falls.

Be prepared to study data measured on an interval scale using non-parametric techniques if it is skewed. Too often unjustified conclusions are drawn from studying skewed data, or by the comparison of two small sample means of widely differing variance.

When you are preparing data for publication, do remember to state the statistical methods which you have used. This will allow readers to judge for themselves the validity (or otherwise) of your conclusions.

4. Misunderstanding of the meaning of P

A probability (P) value, however derived, tells you what is the likelihood of your having arrived at that particular result if the Null Hypothesis were tenable. By convention, when the result will have been arrived at less than once in 20 samples, this is said to indicate a significant departure from the Null Hypothesis ($P < 0.05$) *and that is all*. Always remember that you may simply have picked that one sample in twenty, and thus wrongly rejected the Null Hypothesis (Type I error). If the result is of more than academic interest, you may wish to tighten your definition of significance to $P < 0.01$, or even $P < 0.001$. As noted in (3), unless the departure from the Null Hypothesis is large, this will usually necessitate larger samples.

Another, and most important, point is this. With easy access to microcomputers, it is all too easy to punch in data on a large number of variables and request 't test' or 'regression analysis' on all possible combinations of data sets. If your micro performs 60 't' tests on assorted data sets, three of them will, on average, show an apparent departure from the Null Hypothesis at $P < 0.05$. This is the Type I error at work again.

This also happens far too often in relation to the calculation of correlation coefficients, using data matrices with many variables and fairly small sample size, when '$P < 0.05$' will arise on average, once in 20 such calculations. 'Fishing expeditions' of this sort, in which the investigator 'looks to see' if anything is correlated with anything else, reveal, as a general rule, nothing but ignorance on the part of the investigator of what P values mean. Only very rarely will a nugget of information emerge in this way.

5. Predictive indices
As outlined in Chapter 2, these can be very useful tools. Too often though, their producers confuse sensitivity with specificity. Make sure that you can distinguish between them. Having arrived at a predictive index, which is almost invariably done retrospectively, test it out prospectively before rushing into print with it. The literature is littered with abandoned predictive indices, which, when subjected to test, failed to predict anything.

6. Outliers
Just to remind you. There is an accepted procedure (Chapter 2) for dealing with the occasional outlier. It is otherwise quite unjustifiable to omit data points from any form of statistical analysis just because they 'spoil' a pretty pattern, or don't fit in with your pet hypothesis. If a *properly designed* experiment fails to support your hypothesis, change your hypothesis, not the experiment!

7. Causality
Don't confuse statistical and biological significance, especially in relation to causal inferences made on the basis of correlation and regression analysis. This small book is not the place for a discussion of the logic of drawing causal inferences from studies in medicine. An excellent introductory book on the subject is detailed in *Suggested Further Reading*.

This is the point at which an elementary introduction has to stop. If you have grasped the underlying ideas of the normal distribution and deviations from it, the various ways of describing it, and some of the most basic ways of comparing both parametric and non-parametric data sets, then further forays into statistical theory should present no problem. If, in addition, you now have a vague idea about correlation and regression analysis, then the whole field of partial correlations, multiple regression and factor analysis ceases to be quite so daunting. Statistics are a tool, not a master.

"Lies, damned lies, and statistics"

Disraeli

Suggested further reading

1. Bailey, N. T. J. *Statistical Methods in Biology*. London: Hodder and Stoughton.
   An excellent, clearly written, short text book of basic statistics.
2. Rimm, A. A., Hartz, A. J. Kalbfleisch, J. H., Anderson, A. J. & Hoffman, R. G. *Basic Biostatistics in Medicine and Epidemiology*. New York: Appleton–Century–Crofts.
   Another clearly-written and informative text book, with useful information on the collection of epidemiological data.
3. Snedecor, G. W. & Cochrane, W. G. *Statistical Methods*. Iowa State University Press.
   Considerably more detailed. This is a book for those who become genuinely interested in statistical techniques.
4. K. Diem & C. Lentner (eds). *Documenta Geigy-Scientific tables*. Macclesfield: Geigy Pharmaceuticals.
   An invaluable reference source of expanded statistical tables.
5. Blalock, H. M. *Causal inferences in nonexperimental research*. New York: W. W. Norton.
   A fascinating discussion of the logic, and the logical pitfalls, of research.

Glossary of symbols

a	constant term in the equation for the regression line (Equation 36); the intercept on the y axis when $x = 0$
$a, b, c, d, \ldots$	notation for the observed frequencies in contingency tables
b	calculated regression coefficient (Equation 34)
COV	coefficient of variation (Equation 9)
df	degrees of freedom
D	difference in ranks between paired measurements. Used in the calculation of Spearman's ρ (Equation 31)
e	base of natural logarithms; used in the description of the normal curve (Equation 2)
E	the expected frequency in any cell of a contingency table
f	degrees of freedom for a 't' test with unequal variances (Equation 28)
F	variance ratio (Equation 24)
g	number of groups (columns) in a contingency table
χ^2, χ^2_Y	chi squared (Equations 11–15)
μ, μ_T	true population mean of a distribution
n	number of observations in a sample
O, O_b, O_s	observed frequency in any cell of a contingency table; bigger and smaller of such frequencies in Equation 12
p	proportion of the members of a binomially-distributed sample possessing the attribute under study
π	true proportion of the members of a binomially distributed population possessing the attribute under study
P	probability of arriving at any calculated result if the Null Hypothesis is valid

r	calculated correlation coefficient (Equation 33); number of rows in a contingency table
ρ	Spearman's regression coefficient (Equation 31)
s, s_p	standard deviation; standard deviation from the mean for a binomial distribution (Equation 10)
s^2, s_c^2, s_r^2	variance (Equation 4); combined variance for a 't' test with unequal variances (Equation 26); variance about a regression line (Equation 37)
σ, σ_m, σ_T	true population standard deviation of a distribution
SE	standard error of the mean (Equation 8)
Σ	sum of individual measurements
$\Sigma(x - \bar{x})^2$	sum of squares (Equation 5)
t	Student's 't'
u	ratio used in calculating f (Equation 29)
x	individual values in a sample; independent variable in regression analysis
$\bar{x}$	mean of a sample of xs (Equation 3)
y	dependent variable in regression analysis
z, z_T	standard normal distribution with zero mean and standard deviation of 1

Summary guide to equations

Equation 1

$$\text{Median} = \frac{n+1}{2} \text{ th measurement}$$

Measurements are ranked in ascending order of magnitude.

Equation 2

$$y = \frac{1}{\sigma\sqrt{2\pi}} \, e^{\frac{-(x-\mu)^2}{2\sigma^2}}$$

This describes the normal curve in terms of its population mean, μ, and standard deviation, σ. It is not used directly in this book.

Equation 3

$$\bar{x} = \frac{\Sigma x}{n}$$

The *mean* (average) value, $\bar{x}$, of a sample of n measurements of the variable x. Σx is shorthand for: 'The sum of all the individual values of x', i.e. $x_1 + x_2 + x_3 + \ldots + x_n$.

Since samples are frequently used to describe populations, $\bar{x}$ is used as the approximation to the true population mean, μ.

Equation 4

$$s^2 = \frac{\Sigma(x - \bar{x})^2}{n-1}$$

The *variance, s^2,* of a sample is a measure of the scatter about the sample mean, x, and is used as an estimate of the population variance. The sum of squares, $\Sigma(x - \bar{x})^2$, is most easily calculated from:

Equation 5

$$\Sigma(x - \bar{x})^2 = \Sigma x^2 - \frac{(\Sigma x)^2}{n}$$

The *standard deviation, s,* is simply the square root of the variance. 95% of the values in a sample lie within the range ± 1.96 standard deviations from the mean and 99% lie within the range ± 2.58 standard deviations from the mean.

Equation 6

$$z = \frac{x - \bar{x}}{s}$$

Allows the calculation of the ratio between the difference between an individual value of x and the population or large sample mean, $\bar{x}$, and the standard deviation. Using tables of z (Appendix 1) the area under the normal curve covered by the range $(x - \bar{x})$ can then be read off.

Equation 7

$$s_m = \sqrt{\frac{s_m^2}{m}} \quad \text{or} \quad \frac{s_m}{\sqrt{m}} .$$

Estimates the standard deviation of (from) the population mean where each x in the calculation of s_m^2 is itself a sample mean from the study population, and m such samples have been taken.

Equation 8

$$SE = \sqrt{\frac{s^2}{n}} \quad \text{or} \quad \frac{s}{\sqrt{n}}$$

Directly analogous with Equation 7, this allows the calculation of the *sample* standard deviation of (from) the population mean, usually referred to as the *standard error*.

Equation 9

$$COV = \frac{s}{\bar{x}} \times 100$$

The ratio between the standard deviation and the mean is known as the *coefficient of variation*. It is especially useful in quality control work.

Equation 10

$$s_p = \sqrt{\frac{p \times (1 - p)}{n}}$$

Analogous with Equation 8, but relating to the binomial distribution. If $n > 30$, confidence limits can be calculated as for the normal distribution.

Equation 11

$$\chi^2 = \sum \frac{(O - E)^2}{E}$$

Allows us to assess whether the observed (O) frequency of an event departs significantly from that expected (E) on the basis of the Null Hypothesis (Appendix 2). When only two samples are involved, use:

Equation 12

$$\chi^2 = \frac{(O_b - O_s)^2}{n}$$

where n is the total number of observations. Appendix 2 treats χ^2 as though the numbers involved in the calculation were potentially continuous. In fact, since χ^2 is a non-parametric test, they are not, and a *correction for continuity* should usually be made:

Equation 13

$$\chi_Y^2 = \frac{[O_b - O_s) - 1]^2}{n} \text{ or } \sum \frac{[(O - E) - 0.5]^2}{E}$$

which are minor variants of Equations 11 and 12.

Equation 14

$$\chi^2 = \frac{n(ad - bc)^2}{(a + b)(c + d)(a + c)(b + d)}$$

and

Equation 15

$$\chi^2 = \frac{n[(ad - bc) - \frac{1}{2}n]^2}{(a + b)(c + d)(a + c)(b + d)}$$

are the equivalent calculations for the special case of a
2 × 2 *contingency table* without and with the correction for continuity.

Equation 16

$$P_1 = \frac{(a + b)!\,(c + d)!\,(a + c)!\,(b + d)!}{n!\,a!\,b!\,c!\,d!}$$

calculates exact probabilities for a 2 × 2 contingency
table when the sample sizes are too small to justify the
use of χ^2 (expected values <5). It is repeated after
rearrangement to allow for any more extreme probability (see Chapter 4) and is known as *Fisher's exact
test*.

Equation 17

$$z_T = \frac{(\mu_T - T - \frac{1}{2})}{\sigma_T}$$

Allows calculation of z for *ranked* samples greater in
size than those covered in Appendix 5. The calculated
z is then referred as usual to Appendix 1. T is the rank
total T_1 of the numerically smaller sample when the
lower ranks predominate in this sample. Otherwise, T,
μ_T and σ_T are derived from:

Equation 18

$$T = n_1(n_1 + n_2 + 1) - T_1$$

where T_1 is the rank total from the numerically

smaller sample, of size n_1 and n_2 is the sample size of the second sample.

Equation 19

$$\mu_T = \frac{n_1(n_1 + n_2 + 1)}{2}$$

Equation 20

$$\sigma_T = \sqrt{\frac{n_2 \mu}{6}}$$

Equation 21

$$z = \frac{\bar{x} - \mu}{s/\sqrt{n}}$$

Allows us to test whether a *sample* mean, $\bar{x}$, with standard deviation, s, and sample size, n, where n is > 30 differs significantly from the *population* mean. The variable, x, should be normally-distributed. The calculated z is referred to Appendix 1.

Equation 22

$$z = \frac{\bar{x}_1 - \bar{x}_2}{\sqrt{\dfrac{s_1^2}{n_1} + \dfrac{s_2^2}{n_2}}}$$

This is considerably more useful than Equation 22, since the true population mean is frequently unknown. It allows direct assessment of whether *two sample means*, $\bar{x}_1$ and $\bar{x}_2$, having variances s_1^2 and s_2^2, and of sample sizes n_1 and n_2 where both $n > 30$, differ significantly. The variable, x, should be normally distributed in both samples.

Equation 23

$$z = \frac{p_1 - p_2}{\sqrt{\dfrac{p \times (1 - p)}{n_1} + \dfrac{p \times (1 - p)}{n_2}}}$$

Allows us to assess the statistical significance of the

difference between two *proportions* (percentages), p_1 and p_2, where p is the overall proportion and n_1 and n_2 are the two sample sizes. Refer the calculated z to Appendix 1. Because calculations of proportions such as these assume a binomial distribution, this test should not be carried out when either n is $\leqslant 30$. The further p departs from 0.5 in either direction, the bigger the sample sizes should be, and the more caution is required in interpretation of the results.

Equation 24

$$F = \frac{s_1^2}{s_2^2}$$

where s_1^2 is always the bigger of the two variances under investigation. The calculated F is referred to Appendix 6 with $(n_1 - 1)$ and $(n_2 - 1)$ degrees of freedom. This test should always be performed before comparing the mean values of two small samples ($n \leqslant 30$). When F is significant, Student's 't' test should not be used.

Equation 25

$$t = \frac{\bar{x}_1 - \bar{x}_2}{s_c \sqrt{\frac{1}{n_1} + \frac{1}{n_2}}}$$

Known as *Student's 't' test*. This is used to assess the statistical significance of the difference between two sample means, $\bar{x}$, and $\bar{x}_2$, where either or both of n_1 and n_2 are less than or equal to 30, and s_c is a combined standard deviation calculated from:

Equation 26

$$s_c^2 = \frac{\Sigma_1(x - \bar{x}_1)^2 + \Sigma_2(x - \bar{x}_2)^2}{n_1 + n_2 - 2}$$

where the sums of squares have been calculated as in Equation 5. Refer 't' to Appendix 7 with $(n_1 + n_2 - 2)$ df.

Equation 27

$$t = \frac{\bar{x} - \mu}{s/\sqrt{n}}$$

Student's 't' test for *paired* data. The *difference* between each pair of measurements is considered as a new variable, x, with sample mean x and standard deviation, s. This mean is compared with μ, the hypothetical population mean, where $\mu = 0$ on the Null Hypothesis. Refer 't' to Appendix 7 with $(n - 1)$ df where n is the number of *pairs*.

Equation 28

$$f = \frac{1}{\dfrac{u^2}{(n_1 - 1)} + \dfrac{(1 - u)^2}{(n_2 - 1)}}$$

Calculates the appropriate number of degrees of freedom to use when referring a z value as calculated in Equation 22 to Appendix 7 as a consequence of a significant F test in small samples. u is calculated from:

Equation 29

$$u = \frac{s_1^2/n_1}{s_1^2/n_1 + s_2^2/n_2}$$

where s_1^2 and s_2^2 are the two sample variances. u will, of course, always be < 1.

Equation 30

$$\underset{\substack{\text{between}\\\text{treatments}}}{\Sigma(x - \bar{x})^2} = \frac{(\Sigma x_1)^2}{n_1} + \frac{(\Sigma x_2)^2}{n_2} + \ldots$$

$$+ \frac{(\Sigma x_m)^2}{n_m} - \frac{(\Sigma x_T)^2}{n_T}$$

Analysis of variance breaks down the variation found among several (m) samples subjected to different treatments into that inherent in the samples themselves, and that consequential upon the treatment. The total sum of squares is given by Equation 5; Equation

30 permits calculation of the 'between treatment' sums of squares. Simple subtraction then allows the calculation of the 'within sample' sum of squares. The variances 'between treatment' and 'within sample' are then calculated as usual from Equation 4, remembering that the divisor for the 'between treatment' variance is $(m - 1)$ and that for the 'within group' variance is $(n_T - m)$ where n_T is the total number of observations. The F test (Equation 24) then allows assessment of the statistical significance of the observed result.

Equation 31

$$\rho = 1 - \frac{(6 \times \Sigma D^2)}{n(n^2 - 1)}$$

Allows the calculation of *Spearman's* ρ, an *index of association* between n pairs of ranked data, where D is the difference in rank between each pair. ρ can be either $+$ or $-$, a negative value of ρ indicating an inverse association. The calculated ρ is referred to Appendix 8 in relation to the actual number of pairs of data.

Equation 32

$$\Sigma(x - \bar{x})(y - \bar{y}) = \Sigma xy - \frac{(\Sigma x)(\Sigma y)}{n}$$

Analogous with Equation 5, but relating to the product of the x and y variables. Used in the calculation of the *correlation coefficient*, r, as in:

Equation 33

$$r = \frac{\Sigma(x - \bar{x})(y - \bar{y})}{\sqrt{\Sigma(x - \bar{x})^2 \, \Sigma(y - \bar{y})^2}}$$

This should only be calculated where both x and y are approximately normally distributed. It is a measure of association between the two variables. The function r^2 gives an indication of the proportion of the variability in y which could have occurred in relation to changes in x.

Equation 34

$$b = \frac{\Sigma(x - \bar{x})(y - \bar{y})}{\Sigma(x - \bar{x})^2}$$

Used to determine the slope of the linear association between variables x and y, i.e. the amount by which y changes for a unit change in x. It does not assume that x is normally distributed, although y should be. b is known as the *regression coefficient*.

Equation 35

$$a = \bar{y} - b\bar{x}$$

Used to determine the constant term, i.e. the intercept on the y axis when $x = 0$ in the equation:

Equation 36

$$y = a + bx$$

Once the terms a and b have been calculated as above, this equation can be used to determine the average value of y for any given x; three points so determined allow the drawing of a line of best fit on a scattergram of the raw data.

Equation 37

$$s_r^2 = \frac{1}{n - 2} \left\{ (\Sigma y - \bar{y})^2 - \frac{[\Sigma(x - \bar{x})(y - \bar{y})]^2}{\Sigma(x - \bar{x})^2} \right\}$$

Allows the calculation of the variance, and thus of the standard deviation, about the calculated regression line. From this, we can determine whether our calculated regression coefficient, b, differs from the value of zero which would be assigned to it on the Null Hypothesis.

Equation 38

$$SE_b = \frac{s_r}{\sqrt{\Sigma(x - \bar{x})^2}}$$

This allows calculation of the standard error of the

calculated regression coefficient, b, of (from) the true population coefficient. It is used in:

Equation 39

$$t = \frac{b - 0}{s/\Sigma(x - \bar{x})^2}$$

When the number of pairs of data is greater than 30, the result is referred to Appendix 1. Otherwise use Appendix 7, with $n - 2$ degrees of freedom.

Appendices

Appendices 1, 3, 4, 5 and 8 are taken from Appendices 2, 9, 10, 11 and 12 of Rimm, Hartz, Kalbfleisch, Anderson & Hoffman: *Basic Biostatistics in Medicine and Epidemiology* published by Appleton-Century-Crofts, New York, and by permission of the authors and publishers. Appendices 2, 6, 7 and 9 are taken from Tables I, III, IV, V and VI of Fisher & Yates: *Statistical Tables for Biological, Agricultural and Medical Research* published by Longman Group Ltd., London (previously published by Oliver and Boyd Ltd., Edinburgh), and by permission of the authors and publishers.

Appendix 1 Normal Probability Distribution $-3.70 \leq z \leq 0.95$ and Special Quantiles*

Special Quantiles

z	P(Z≤z)	P(Z≥z)	z	P(Z≤z)	P(Z≥z)
-3.719	0.0001	0.9999	0.000	0.50	0.50
-3.291	0.0005	0.9995	0.126	0.55	0.45
-3.090	0.001	0.999	0.253	0.60	0.40
-2.576	0.005	0.995	0.385	0.65	0.35
-2.326	0.010	0.990	0.524	0.70	0.30
-1.960	0.025	0.975	0.674	0.75	0.25
-1.645	0.05	0.95	0.842	0.80	0.20
-1.282	0.10	0.90	1.036	0.85	0.15
-1.036	0.15	0.85	1.282	0.90	0.10
-0.842	0.20	0.80	1.645	0.95	0.05
-0.674	0.25	0.75	1.960	0.975	0.025
-0.524	0.30	0.70	2.326	0.990	0.010
-0.385	0.35	0.65	2.576	0.995	0.005
-0.253	0.40	0.60	3.090	0.999	0.001
-0.126	0.45	0.55	3.291	0.9995	0.0005

Distribution

z	P(Z≤z)	P(Z≥z)
-3.70	0.0001	0.9999
-3.60	0.0002	0.9998
-3.50	0.0002	0.9998
-3.40	0.0003	0.9997
-3.30	0.0005	0.9995
-3.25	0.0006	0.9994
-3.20	0.0007	0.9993
-3.15	0.0008	0.9992
-3.10	0.0010	0.9990
-3.05	0.0011	0.9989
-3.00	0.0013	0.9987
-2.95	0.0016	0.9984
-2.90	0.0019	0.9981
-2.85	0.0022	0.9978
-2.80	0.0026	0.9974
-2.75	0.0030	0.9970
-2.70	0.0035	0.9965
-2.65	0.0040	0.9960
-2.60	0.0047	0.9953
-2.55	0.0054	0.9946
-2.50	0.0062	0.9938
-2.45	0.0071	0.9929
-2.40	0.0082	0.9918
-2.35	0.0094	0.9906
-2.30	0.0107	0.9893
-2.25	0.0122	0.9878
-2.20	0.0139	0.9861
-2.15	0.0158	0.9842
-2.10	0.0179	0.9821
-2.05	0.0202	0.9798
-2.00	0.0228	0.9772
-1.95	0.0256	0.9744
-1.90	0.0287	0.9713
-1.85	0.0322	0.9678
-1.80	0.0359	0.9641
-1.75	0.0401	0.9599
-1.70	0.0446	0.9554
-1.65	0.0495	0.9505
-1.60	0.0548	0.9452
-1.55	0.0606	0.9394
-1.50	0.0668	0.9332
-1.45	0.0735	0.9265
-1.40	0.0808	0.9192
-1.35	0.0885	0.9115
-1.30	0.0968	0.9032
-1.25	0.1056	0.8944
-1.20	0.1151	0.8849
-1.15	0.1251	0.8749
-1.10	0.1357	0.8643
-1.05	0.1469	0.8531
-1.00	0.1587	0.8413
-0.95	0.1711	0.8289
-0.90	0.1841	0.8159
-0.85	0.1977	0.8023
-0.80	0.2119	0.7881
-0.75	0.2266	0.7734
-0.70	0.2420	0.7580
-0.65	0.2578	0.7422
-0.60	0.2743	0.7257
-0.55	0.2912	0.7088
-0.50	0.3085	0.6915
-0.45	0.3264	0.6736
-0.40	0.3446	0.6554
-0.35	0.3632	0.6368
-0.30	0.3821	0.6179
-0.25	0.4013	0.5987
-0.20	0.4207	0.5793
-0.15	0.4404	0.5596
-0.10	0.4602	0.5398
-0.05	0.4801	0.5199
0.00	0.5000	0.5000
0.05	0.5199	0.4801
0.10	0.5398	0.4602
0.15	0.5596	0.4404
0.20	0.5793	0.4207
0.25	0.5987	0.4013
0.30	0.6179	0.3821
0.35	0.6368	0.3632
0.40	0.6554	0.3446
0.45	0.6736	0.3264
0.50	0.6915	0.3085
0.55	0.7088	0.2912
0.60	0.7257	0.2743
0.65	0.7422	0.2578
0.70	0.7580	0.2420
0.75	0.7734	0.2266
0.80	0.7881	0.2119
0.85	0.8023	0.1977
0.90	0.8159	0.1841
0.95	0.8289	0.1711
1.00	0.8413	0.1587
1.05	0.8531	0.1469
1.10	0.8643	0.1357
1.15	0.8749	0.1251
1.20	0.8849	0.1151
1.25	0.8944	0.1056
1.30	0.9032	0.0968
1.35	0.9115	0.0885
1.40	0.9192	0.0808
1.45	0.9265	0.0735
1.50	0.9332	0.0668
1.55	0.9394	0.0606
1.60	0.9452	0.0548
1.65	0.9505	0.0495
1.70	0.9554	0.0446
1.75	0.9599	0.0401
1.80	0.9641	0.0359
1.85	0.9678	0.0322
1.90	0.9713	0.0287
1.95	0.9744	0.0256
2.00	0.9772	0.0228
2.05	0.9798	0.0202
2.10	0.9821	0.0179
2.15	0.9842	0.0158
2.20	0.9861	0.0139
2.25	0.9878	0.0122
2.30	0.9893	0.0107
2.35	0.9906	0.0094
2.40	0.9918	0.0082
2.45	0.9929	0.0071
2.50	0.9938	0.0062
2.55	0.9946	0.0054
2.60	0.9953	0.0047
2.65	0.9960	0.0040
2.70	0.9965	0.0035
2.75	0.9970	0.0030
2.80	0.9974	0.0026
2.85	0.9978	0.0022
2.90	0.9981	0.0019
2.95	0.9984	0.0016
3.00	0.9987	0.0013
3.05	0.9989	0.0011
3.10	0.9990	0.0010
3.15	0.9992	0.0008
3.20	0.9993	0.0007
3.25	0.9994	0.0006
3.30	0.9995	0.0005
3.40	0.9997	0.0003
3.50	0.9998	0.0002
3.60	0.9998	0.0002
3.70	0.9999	0.0001

* $P(Z \leq z)$ column gives area to the left of z; $P(Z \geq z)$ column gives area to the right of z.

Appendix 2   The χ^2 distribution

Degrees of freedom	Value of P				
	0.99	0.95	0.05	0.01	0.001
1	0.000157	0.00393	3.841	6.635	10.83
2	0.0201	0.103	5.991	9.210	13.82
3	0.115	0.352	7.815	11.34	16.27
4	0.297	0.711	9.488	13.28	18.47
5	0.554	1.145	11.07	15.09	20.51
6	0.872	1.635	12.59	16.81	22.46
7	1.239	2.167	14.07	18.48	24.32
8	1.646	2.733	15.51	20.09	26.13
9	2.088	3.325	16.92	21.67	27.88
10	2.558	3.940	18.31	23.21	29.59
11	3.053	4.575	19.68	24.72	31.26
12	3.571	5.226	21.03	26.22	32.91
13	4.107	5.892	22.36	27.69	34.53
14	4.660	6.571	23.68	29.14	36.12
15	5.229	7.261	25.00	30.58	37.70
16	5.812	7.962	26.30	32.00	39.25
17	6.408	8.672	27.59	33.41	40.79
18	7.015	9.390	28.87	34.81	42.31
19	7.633	10.12	30.14	36.19	43.82
20	8.260	10.85	31.41	37.57	45.31
21	8.897	11.59	32.67	38.93	46.80
22	9.542	12.34	33.92	40.29	48.27
23	10.20	13.09	35.17	41.64	49.73
24	10.86	13.85	36.42	42.98	51.18
25	11.52	14.61	37.65	44.31	52.62
26	12.20	15.38	38.89	45.64	54.05
27	12.88	16.15	40.11	46.96	55.48
28	13.56	16.93	41.34	48.28	56.89
29	14.26	17.71	42.56	49.59	58.30
30	14.95	18.49	43.77	50.89	59.70

The table gives the percentage points most frequently required for significance tests based on χ^2. Thus the probability of observing a χ^2 with 5 degrees of freedom *greater* in value than 11.07 is 0.05 or 5%. Again, the probability of observing a χ^2 with 5 degrees of freedom *smaller* in value than 0.554 is $1 - 0.99 = 0.01$ or 1%.

Appendix 3 Critical Values of *n* for the Sign Test

n	1%	5%	10%	25%	n	1%	5%	10%	25%
1					46	13	15	16	18
2					47	14	16	17	19
3				0	48	14	16	17	19
4				0	49	15	17	18	19
5			0	0	50	15	17	18	20
6		0	0	1	51	15	18	19	20
7		0	0	1	52	16	18	19	21
8	0	0	1	1	53	16	18	20	21
9	0	1	1	2	54	17	19	20	22
10	0	1	1	2	55	17	19	20	22
11	0	1	2	3	56	17	20	21	23
12	1	2	2	3	57	18	20	21	23
13	1	2	3	3	58	18	21	22	24
14	1	2	3	4	59	19	21	22	24
15	2	3	3	4	60	19	21	23	25
16	2	3	4	5	61	20	22	23	25
17	2	4	4	5	62	20	22	24	25
18	3	4	5	6	63	20	23	24	26
19	2	4	5	6	64	21	23	24	26
20	3	5	5	6	65	21	24	25	27
21	4	5	6	7	66	22	24	25	27
22	4	5	6	7	67	22	25	26	28
23	4	6	7	8	68	22	25	26	28
24	5	6	7	8	69	23	25	27	29
25	5	7	7	9	70	23	26	27	29
26	6	7	8	9	71	24	26	28	30
27	6	7	8	10	72	24	27	28	30
28	6	8	9	10	73	25	27	28	31
29	7	8	9	10	74	25	28	29	31
30	7	9	10	11	75	25	28	29	32
31	7	9	10	11	76	26	28	30	32
32	8	9	10	12	77	26	29	30	32
33	8	10	11	12	78	27	29	31	33
34	9	10	11	13	79	27	30	31	33
35	9	11	12	13	80	28	30	32	34
36	9	11	12	14	81	28	31	32	34
37	10	12	13	14	82	28	31	33	35
38	10	12	13	14	83	29	32	33	35
39	11	12	13	15	84	29	32	33	36
40	11	13	14	15	85	30	32	34	36
41	11	13	14	16	86	30	33	34	37
42	12	14	15	16	87	31	33	35	37
43	12	14	15	17	88	31	34	35	38
44	13	15	16	17	89	31	34	36	38
45	13	15	16	18	90	32	35	36	39

Appendix 4   Critical Range of T^* for the Wilcoxon Signed Rank Test

	Level of Significance for Two-Tailed Test			
N	0.10	0.05	0.02	0.01
5	0–15			
6	2–19	0–21		
7	3–25	2–26	0–28	
8	5–31	3–33	1–35	0–36
9	8–37	5–40	3–42	1–44
10	10–45	8–47	5–50	3–52
11	13–53	10–56	7–59	5–61
12	17–61	13–65	9–69	7–71
13	21–70	17–74	12–79	9–82
14	25–80	21–84	15–90	12–93
15	30–90	25–95	19–101	15–105
16	35–101	29–107	23–113	19–117
17	41–112	34–119	28–125	23–130
18	47–124	40–131	32–129	27–144
19	53–137	46–144	37–153	32–158
20	60–150	52–158	43–167	37–173
21	67–164	58–173	49–182	42–189
22	75–178	66–187	55–198	48–205
23	83–193	73–203	62–214	54–222
24	91–209	81–219	69–231	61–239
25	100–225	89–236	76–249	68–257
26	110–241	98–253	84–267	75–276
27	119–259	107–271	92–286	83–295
28	130–276	116–290	101–305	91–315
29	140–295	126–309	110–326	100–335
30	151–314	137–328	120–345	109–356
31	163–333	147–349	130–366	118–378
32	175–353	159–369	140–388	128–400
33	187–374	170–391	151–410	138–423
34	200–395	182–413	162–433	148–447
35	213–417	195–435	173–457	159–471
36	227–439	208–458	185–481	171–495
37	241–462	221–482	198–505	182–521
38	256–485	235–506	211–530	194–547
39	271–509	249–531	224–556	207–573
40	286–534	264–556	238–582	220–600
41	302–559	279–582	252–609	233–628
42	319–584	294–609	266–637	247–656
43	336–610	310–636	281–665	261–685
44	353–637	327–663	296–694	276–714
45	371–664	343–692	312–723	291–744
46	389–692	361–720	328–753	307–774
47	407–721	378–750	345–783	322–806
48	426–750	396–780	362–814	339–837
49	446–779	415–810	379–846	335–870
50	466–809	434–841	397–878	373–902

* The Symbol T denotes the sum of ranks associated with differences that are all of the same sign. For any given N (number of ranked differences), the obtained T is significant at a given level if it is equal to or less than the smaller value shown in the table or equal to or greater than the larger value shown in the table.

Appendix 5 Critical Range of Rank Sums $T*$ (Two-Tailed Alternative)

Critical Range for the following n_1:

n_2	P	2	3	4	5	6	7	8	9	10	11	12	13	14
4	0.05			10–26	16–34	23–43	31–53	40–64	49–77	60–90	72–104	85–119	99–135	114–152
	0.01					21–45	28–56	37–67	46–80	57–93	68–108	81–123	94–140	109–157
5	0.05			11–29	17–38	24–48	33–58	42–70	52–83	63–97	75–112	89–127	103–144	118–162
	0.01				15–40	22–50	29–62	38–74	48–87	59–101	71–116	84–132	98–149	112–168
6	0.05			12–32	18–42	26–52	34–64	44–76	55–89	66–104	79–119	92–136	107–153	122–172
	0.01			10–34	16–44	23–55	31–67	40–80	50–94	61–109	73–125	87–141	101–159	116–178
7	0.05			13–35	20–45	27–57	36–69	46–82	57–96	69–111	82–127	96–144	111–162	127–181
	0.01			10–38	16–49	24–60	32–73	42–86	52–101	64–116	76–133	90–150	104–169	120–188
8	0.05	3–19	8–28	14–38	21–49	29–61	38–74	49–87	60–102	72–118	85–135	100–152	115–171	131–191
	0.01			11–41	17–53	25–65	34–78	43–93	54–108	66–124	79–141	93–159	108–178	123–199
9	0.05	3–21	8–31	14–42	22–53	31–65	40–79	51–93	62–109	75–125	89–142	104–160	119–180	136–200
	0.01		6–33	11–45	18–57	26–70	35–84	45–99	56–115	68–132	82–149	96–168	111–188	127–209
10	0.05	3–23	9–36	15–45	23–57	32–70	42–84	53–99	65–115	78–132	92–150	107–169	124–188	141–209
	0.01		6–36	12–48	19–61	27–75	37–89	47–105	58–122	71–139	84–158	99–177	115–197	131–219
11	0.05	4–24	10–38	16–48	24–61	34–74	44–89	55–105	68–121	81–139	96–157	111–177	128–197	145–219
	0.01		6–39	12–52	20–65	28–80	38–95	49–111	61–128	73–147	87–166	102–186	118–207	135–229
12	0.05	4–26	10–41	17–51	26–64	35–79	46–94	58–110	71–127	84–146	99–165	115–185	132–206	150–228
	0.01		7–41	13–55	21–69	30–84	40–100	51–117	63–135	76–154	90–174	105–195	122–216	139–239
13	0.05	4–28	11–43	18–54	27–68	37–83	48–99	60–116	73–134	88–152	103–172	119–193	136–215	155–237
	0.01		7–44	13–59	22–73	31–89	41–106	53–123	65–142	79–161	93–182	109–203	125–226	143–249
14	0.05	4–30	11–46	19–57	28–72	38–88	50–104	62–122	76–140	91–159	106–180	123–201	141–223	160–246
	0.01		7–47	14–62	22–78	32–94	43–111	54–130	67–149	81–169	96–190	112–212	129–235	147–259
15	0.05	4–32	12–48	20–60	29–76	40–92	52–109	65–127	79–146	94–166	110–187	127–209	145–232	164–256
	0.01		8–49	15–65	23–82	33–99	44–117	56–136	69–156	84–176	99–198	115–221	133–244	151–269
16	0.05	4–34	12–51	21–63	30–80	42–96	54–114	67–133	82–152	97–173	113–195	131–217	150–240	169–265
	0.01		8–52	15–69	24–86	34–104	46–122	58–142	72–162	86–184	102–206	119–229	136–254	155–279
17	0.05	5–35	13–53	21–67	32–83	43–101	56–119	70–138	84–159	100–180	117–202	135–225	154–249	174–274
	0.01		8–55	16–72	25–90	36–108	47–128	60–148	74–169	89–191	105–214	122–238	140–263	160–288
18	0.05	5–37	13–56	22–70	33–87	45–105	58–124	72–144	87–165	103–187	121–209	139–233	159–257	179–283
	0.01		8–58	16–76	26–94	37–113	49–133	62–154	76–176	92–198	108–222	125–247	144–272	164–298
19	0.05	5–39		23–73	34–91	46–110	60–129	74–150	90–171	107–193	124–217	143–241	163–266	184–299
	0.01	3–41	9–60	17–79	27–98	38–118	50–139	64–160	78–183	94–206	111–230	129–255	148–281	168–308

* The symbol T denotes the sum of ranks associated with the smaller sample (n_1). The obtained T is significant at a given level if it is equal to or less than the smaller value shown in the table or equal to or greater than the larger value shown in the table value.

Appendix 6 5° points of variance-ratio (F) distribution

f_2 \ f_1	1	2	3	4	5	6	7	8	9	10	12	15	20	30	∞
1	161.4	199.5	215.7	224.6	230.2	234.0	236.8	238.9	240.5	241.9	243.9	245.9	248.0	250.1	254.3
2	18.51	19.00	19.16	19.25	19.30	19.33	19.35	19.37	19.38	19.40	19.41	19.43	19.45	19.46	19.50
3	10.13	9.55	9.28	9.12	9.01	8.94	8.89	8.85	8.81	8.79	8.74	8.70	8.66	8.62	8.53
4	7.71	6.94	6.59	6.39	6.26	6.16	6.09	6.04	6.00	5.96	5.91	5.86	5.80	5.75	5.63
5	6.61	5.79	5.41	5.19	5.05	4.95	4.88	4.82	4.77	4.74	4.68	4.62	4.56	4.50	4.36
6	5.99	5.14	4.76	4.53	4.39	4.28	4.21	4.15	4.10	4.06	4.00	3.94	3.87	3.81	3.67
7	5.59	4.74	4.35	4.12	3.97	3.87	3.79	3.73	3.68	3.64	3.57	3.51	3.44	3.38	3.23
8	5.32	4.46	4.07	3.84	3.69	3.58	3.50	3.44	3.39	3.35	3.28	3.22	3.15	3.08	2.93
9	5.12	4.26	3.86	3.63	3.48	3.37	3.29	3.23	3.18	3.14	3.07	3.01	2.94	2.86	2.71
10	4.96	4.10	3.71	3.48	3.33	3.22	3.14	3.07	3.02	2.98	2.91	2.85	2.77	2.70	2.54
11	4.84	3.98	3.59	3.36	3.20	3.09	3.01	2.95	2.90	2.85	2.79	2.72	2.65	2.57	2.40
12	4.75	3.89	3.49	3.26	3.11	3.00	2.91	2.85	2.80	2.75	2.69	2.62	2.54	2.47	2.30
13	4.67	3.81	3.41	3.18	3.03	2.92	2.83	2.77	2.71	2.67	2.60	2.53	2.46	2.38	2.21
14	4.60	3.74	3.34	3.11	2.96	2.85	2.76	2.70	2.65	2.60	2.53	2.46	2.39	2.31	2.13
15	4.54	3.68	3.29	3.06	2.90	2.79	2.71	2.64	2.59	2.54	2.48	2.40	2.33	2.25	2.07
16	4.49	3.63	3.24	3.01	2.85	2.74	2.66	2.59	2.54	2.49	2.42	2.35	2.28	2.19	2.01
17	4.45	3.59	3.20	2.96	2.81	2.70	2.61	2.55	2.49	2.45	2.38	2.31	2.23	2.15	1.96
18	4.41	3.55	3.16	2.93	2.77	2.66	2.58	2.51	2.46	2.41	2.34	2.27	2.19	2.11	1.92
19	4.38	3.52	3.13	2.90	2.74	2.63	2.54	2.48	2.42	2.38	2.31	2.23	2.16	2.07	1.88
20	4.35	3.49	3.10	2.87	2.71	2.60	2.51	2.45	2.39	2.35	2.28	2.20	2.12	2.04	1.84

Appendix 6 (*continued*) 5° points of variance-ratio (*F*) distribution

f_2 \ f_1	1	2	3	4	5	6	7	8	9	10	12	15	20	30	∞
21	4.32	3.47	3.07	2.84	2.68	2.57	2.49	2.42	2.37	2.32	2.25	2.18	2.10	2.01	1.81
22	4.30	3.44	3.05	2.82	2.66	2.55	2.46	2.40	2.34	2.30	2.23	2.15	2.07	1.98	1.78
23	4.28	3.42	3.03	2.80	2.64	2.53	2.44	2.37	2.32	2.27	2.20	2.13	2.05	1.96	1.76
24	4.26	3.40	3.01	2.78	2.62	2.51	2.42	2.36	2.30	2.25	2.18	2.11	2.03	1.94	1.73
25	4.24	3.39	2.99	2.76	2.60	2.49	2.40	2.34	2.28	2.24	2.16	2.09	2.01	1.92	1.71
26	4.23	3.37	2.98	2.74	2.59	2.47	2.39	2.32	2.27	2.22	2.15	2.07	1.99	1.90	1.69
27	4.21	3.35	2.96	2.73	2.57	2.46	2.37	2.31	2.25	2.20	2.13	2.06	1.97	1.88	1.67
28	4.20	3.34	2.95	2.71	2.56	2.45	2.36	2.29	2.24	2.19	2.12	2.04	1.96	1.87	1.65
29	4.18	3.33	2.93	2.70	2.55	2.43	2.35	2.28	2.22	2.18	2.10	2.03	1.94	1.85	1.64
30	4.17	3.32	2.92	2.69	2.53	2.42	2.33	2.27	2.21	2.16	2.09	2.01	1.93	1.84	1.62
40	4.08	3.23	2.84	2.61	2.45	2.34	2.25	2.18	2.12	2.08	2.00	1.92	1.84	1.74	1.51
60	4.00	3.15	2.76	2.53	2.37	2.25	2.17	2.10	2.04	1.99	1.92	1.84	1.75	1.65	1.39
120	3.92	3.07	2.68	2.45	2.29	2.17	2.09	2.02	1.96	1.91	1.83	1.75	1.66	1.55	1.25
∞	3.84	3.00	2.60	2.37	2.21	2.10	2.01	1.94	1.88	1.83	1.75	1.67	1.57	1.46	1.00

The table gives the 5° points of the distribution of the variance-ratio, $F = s_1^2/s_1^2$, where the numerator and denominator have f_1 and f_2 degrees of freedom respectively. Thus if $f_1 = 7$ and $f_2 = 15$, the probability that the observed value of F is *greater* than 2.71 is exactly 0.05 or 5°.

Appendix 6 (*continued*) 1° points of variance-ratio (*F*) distribution

f_2 \ f_1	1	2	3	4	5	6	7	8	9	10	12	15	20	30	∞
1	4052	4999	5403	5625	5764	5859	5928	5982	6022	6056	6106	6157	6209	6261	6366
2	98.50	99.00	99.17	99.25	99.30	99.33	99.36	99.37	99.39	99.40	99.42	99.43	99.45	99.47	99.0
3	34.12	30.82	29.46	28.71	28.24	27.91	27.67	27.49	27.35	27.23	27.05	26.87	26.69	26.50	26.13
4	21.20	18.00	16.69	15.98	15.52	15.21	14.98	14.80	14.66	14.55	14.37	14.20	14.02	13.84	13.46
5	16.26	13.27	12.06	11.39	10.97	10.67	10.46	10.29	10.16	10.05	9.89	9.72	9.55	9.38	9.02
6	13.75	10.92	9.78	9.15	8.75	8.47	8.26	8.10	7.98	7.87	7.72	7.56	7.40	7.23	6.88
7	12.25	9.5	8.45	7.85	7.46	7.19	6.99	6.84	6.72	6.62	6.47	6.31	6.16	5.99	5.65
8	11.26	8.65	7.59	7.01	6.63	6.37	6.18	6.03	5.91	5.81	5.67	5.52	5.36	5.20	4.86
9	10.56	8.02	6.99	6.42	6.06	5.80	5.61	5.47	5.35	5.26	5.11	4.96	4.81	4.65	4.31
10	10.04	7.56	6.55	5.99	5.64	5.39	5.20	5.06	4.94	4.85	4.71	4.56	4.41	4.25	.3.91
11	9.65	7.21	6.22	5.67	5.32	5.07	4.89	4.74	4.63	4.54	4.40	4.25	4.10	3.94	3.60
12	9.33	6.93	5.95	5.41	5.06	4.82	4.64	4.50	4.39	4.30	4.16	4.01	3.86	3.70	3.36
13	9.07	6.70	5.74	5.21	4.86	4.62	4.44	4.30	4.19	4.10	3.96	3.82	3.66	3.51	3.17
14	8.86	6.51	5.56	5.04	4.69	4.46	4.28	4.14	4.03	3.94	3.80	3.66	3.51	3.35	3.00
15	8.68	6.36	5.42	4.89	4.56	4.32	4.14	4.00	3.89	3.80	3.67	3.52	3.37	3.21	2.87
16	8.53	6.23	5.29	4.77	4.44	4.20	4.03	3.89	3.78	3.69	3.55	3.41	3.26	3.10	2.75
17	8.40	6.11	5.18	4.67	4.34	4.10	3.93	3.79	3.68	3.59	3.46	3.31	3.16	3.00	2.65
18	8.29	6.01	5.09	4.58	4.25	4.01	3.84	3.71	3.60	3.51	3.37	3.23	3.08	2.92	2.57
19	8.18	5.93	5.01	4.50	4.17	3.94	3.77	3.63	3.52	3.43	3.30	3.15	3.00	2.84	2.49
20	8.10	5.85	4.94	4.43	4.10	3.87	3.70	3.56	3.46	3.37	3.23	3.09	2.94	2.78	2.42

Appendix 6 (*continued*) 1° points of variance-ratio (*F*) distribution

f_2 \ f_1	1	2	3	4	5	6	7	8	9	10	12	15	20	30	∞
21	8.02	5.78	4.87	4.37	4.04	3.81	3.64	3.51	3.40	3.31	3.17	3.03	2.88	2.72	2.36
22	7.95	5.72	4.82	4.31	3.99	3.76	3.59	3.45	3.35	3.26	3.12	2.98	2.83	2.67	2.31
23	7.88	5.66	4.76	4.26	3.94	3.71	3.54	3.41	3.30	3.21	3.07	2.93	2.78	2.62	2.26
24	7.82	5.61	4.72	4.22	3.90	3.67	3.50	3.36	3.26	3.17	3.03	2.89	2.74	2.58	2.21
25	7.77	5.57	4.68	4.18	3.85	3.63	3.46	3.32	3.22	3.13	2.99	2.85	2.70	2.54	2.17
26	7.72	5.53	4.64	4.14	3.82	3.59	3.42	3.29	3.18	3.09	2.96	2.81	2.66	2.50	2.13
27	7.68	5.49	4.60	4.11	3.78	3.56	3.39	3.26	3.15	3.06	2.93	2.78	2.63	2.47	2.10
28	7.64	5.45	4.57	4.07	3.75	3.53	3.36	3.23	3.12	3.03	2.90	2.75	2.60	2.44	2.06
29	7.60	5.42	4.54	4.04	3.73	3.50	3.33	3.20	3.09	3.00	2.87	2.73	2.57	2.41	2.03
30	7.56	5.39	4.51	4.02	3.70	3.47	3.30	3.17	3.07	2.98	2.84	2.70	2.55	2.39	2.01
40	7.31	5.18	4.31	3.83	3.51	3.29	3.12	2.99	2.89	2.80	2.66	2.52	2.37	2.20	1.80
60	7.08	4.98	4.13	3.65	3.34	3.12	2.95	2.82	2.72	2.63	2.50	2.35	2.20	2.03	1.60
120	6.85	4.79	3.95	3.48	3.17	2.96	2.79	2.66	2.56	2.47	2.34	2.19	2.03	1.86	1.38
∞	6.63	4.61	3.78	3.32	3.02	2.80	2.64	2.51	2.41	2.32	2.18	2.04	1.88	1.70	1.00

The table gives 1° points of the distribution of the variance-ratio, $F = s_1^2/s_2^2$, where the numerator and denominator have f_1 and f_2 degrees of freedom respectively.
Thus if $f_1 = 7$ and $f_2 = 15$, the probability that the observed value of *F* is *greater* than 4.14 is exactly 0.01 or 1°.

Appendix 7 'Student's' t-distribution

Degrees of freedom	Value of P					
	0.10	0.05	0.02	0.01	0.002	0.001
1	6.314	12.71	31.82	63.66	318.3	636.6
2	2.920	4.303	6.965	9.925	22.33	31.60
3	2.353	3.182	4.541	5.841	10.21	12.92
4	2.132	2.776	3.747	4.604	7.173	8.610
5	2.015	2.571	3.365	4.032	5.893	6.869
6	1.943	2.447	3.143	3.707	5.208	5.959
7	1.895	2.365	2.998	3.499	4.785	5.408
8	1.860	2.306	2.896	3.355	4.501	5.041
9	1.833	2.262	2.821	3.250	4.297	4.781
10	1.812	2.228	2.764	3.169	4.144	4.587
11	1.796	2.201	2.718	3.106	4.025	4.437
12	1.782	2.179	2.681	3.055	3.930	4.318
13	1.771	2.160	2.650	3.012	3.852	4.221
14	1.761	2.145	2.624	2.977	3.787	4.140
15	1.753	2.131	2.602	2.947	3.733	4.073
16	1.746	2.120	2.583	2.921	3.686	4.015
17	1.740	2.110	2.567	2.898	3.646	3.965
18	1.734	2.101	2.552	2.878	3.610	3.922
19	1.729	2.093	2.539	2.861	3.579	3.883
20	1.725	2.086	2.528	2.845	3.552	3.850
21	1.721	2.080	2.518	2.831	3.527	3.819
22	1.717	2.074	2.508	2.819	3.505	3.792
23	1.714	2.069	2.500	2.807	3.485	3.767
24	1.711	2.064	2.492	2.797	3.467	3.745
25	1.708	2.060	2.485	2.787	3.450	3.725
26	1.706	2.056	2.479	2.779	3.435	3.707
27	1.703	2.052	2.473	2.771	3.421	3.690
28	1.701	2.048	2.467	2.763	3.408	3.674
29	1.699	2.045	2.462	2.756	3.396	3.659
30	1.697	2.042	2.457	2.750	3.385	3.646

The table gives the percentage points most frequently required for significance tests and confidence limits based on 'Student's' t-distribution. Thus the probability of observing a value of t, with 10 degrees of freedom, greater in *absolute value* than 3.169 (i.e. < -3.169 or $> +3.169$) is exactly 0.01 or 1%.

Appendix 8 Significance Levels of ρ the Spearman Rank Order Correlation Coefficient

| n^* | Level of significance for two-tailed test | | | |
	0.10	0.05	0.02	0.01
5	0.900	1.000	1.000	—
6	0.829	0.886	0.943	1.000
7	0.714	0.786	0.893	0.929
8	0.643	0.738	0.833	0.881
9	0.600	0.683	0.783	0.833
10	0.564	0.648	0.746	0.794
12	0.506	0.591	0.712	0.777
14	0.456	0.544	0.645	0.715
16	0.425	0.506	0.601	0.665
18	0.399	0.475	0.564	0.625
20	0.377	0.450	0.534	0.591
22	0.359	0.428	0.508	0.562
24	0.343	0.409	0.485	0.537
26	0.329	0.392	0.465	0.515
28	0.317	0.377	0.448	0.496
30	0.306	0.364	0.432	0.478

* n = number of pairs. When $n > 30$, refer ρ to Appendix 9.

Appendix 9   The correlation coefficient

Degrees of freedom $(n - 2)$	Value of P				
	0.10	0.05	0.02	0.01	0.001
1	0.9877	0.99692	0.99951	0.99988	0.9999988
2	0.9000	0.9500	0.9800	0.9900	0.9990
3	0.805	0.878	0.9343	0.9587	0.9911
4	0.729	0.811	0.882	0.9172	0.9741
5	0.669	0.754	0.833	0.875	0.9509
6	0.621	0.707	0.789	0.834	0.9249
7	0.582	0.666	0.750	0.798	0.898
8	0.549	0.632	0.715	0.765	0.872
9	0.521	0.602	0.685	0.735	0.847
10	0.497	0.576	0.658	0.708	0.823
11	0.476	0.553	0.634	0.684	0.801
12	0.457	0.532	0.612	0.661	0.780
13	0.441	0.514	0.592	0.641	0.760
14	0.426	0.497	0.574	0.623	0.742
15	0.412	0.482	0.558	0.606	0.725
16	0.400	0.468	0.543	0.590	0.708
17	0.389	0.456	0.529	0.575	0.693
18	0.378	0.444	0.516	0.561	0.679
19	0.369	0.433	0.503	0.549	0.665
20	0.360	0.423	0.492	0.537	0.652
25	0.323	0.381	0.445	0.487	0.597
30	0.296	0.349	0.409	0.449	0.554
35	0.275	0.325	0.381	0.418	0.519
40	0.257	0.304	0.358	0.393	0.490
45	0.243	0.288	0.338	0.372	0.465
50	0.231	0.273	0.322	0.354	0.443
60	0.211	0.250	0.295	0.325	0.408
70	0.195	0.232	0.274	0.302	0.380
80	0.183	0.217	0.257	0.283	0.357
90	0.173	0.205	0.242	0.267	0.338
100	0.164	0.195	0.230	0.254	0.321

The table gives percentage points for the distribution of the estimated correlation coefficient r when the true value ρ is zero. Thus when there are 10 degrees of freedom (i.e. in samples of 12) the probability of observing an r greater in *absolute value* than 0.576 (i.e. < -0.576 or $> +0.576$) is 0.05 or 5%.

Index

Accuracy, 2
Adjustment (standardization) of rates, 7–8
Analysis of variance, 71, 85–88
  comparison of means, 87, 88
  table of, 86–87
Association, 50, 91, 92, 95, 98, 101, 102
  negative (inverse), 94, 102
  of non-parametric or non-normally distributed variables, 91–94, 102
  see also Chi-squared (χ^2); Spearman's rank correlation coefficient (ρ) positive; Correlation; Regression analysis
Average, 12

Best fit, line of, 94, 99–100, 102
Bias, 3
Binomial distribution, *see* Distribution, binomial
Biological significance, 5, 91, 108

Calculators, use of, 15, 73, 74, 88
Causality, 91, 102, 108
Chi-squared (χ^2), 36–41, 42, 48–52, 59
  calculation of, 37, 47, 48, 51, 92
    expected values, 36, 38, 47, 49, 92
    observed values, 36–37
    shortcut, 47
  degrees of freedom, 38, 41, 42, 50, 92
  for contingency tables, 48–52, 59
  for 2 × 2 tables, 51–52, 59
  goodness of fit, 38, 39–41
  test for association, 50, 91–92, 102
  Yates' correction, 48, 51, 59
Classification of diseases, 19–21, 28
Coefficient of variation, 24–25, 28
Computers, 96, 101, 107
Concordance, 93
  negative, 94
Confidence intervals, 24, 26, 28, 33, 42
Contingency tables, 48–53, 59
  collapsing groups/rows, 38, 40, 50, 59
  degrees of freedom, 50
  expected values, 49, 50, 92
  groups (columns), 38, 49, 50
  rows, 49, 50
  2 × 2, 51–52, 59
  see also Chi-squared (χ^2), for contingency tables

Continuity, correction for, 48, 51, 58
  see also Chi-squared, Yates' correction
Control data, 55, 69, 106
Correlation, 91, 93–97, 102
  assumptions, 94
  coefficient of (r), 96–97, 102, 107
    degrees of freedom of, 97, 102
    r^2, use of, 97, 102
  negative, 94, 102
  partial, 97
  positive, 94, 102
Covariance, 96
Crude rates, 6, 7
Cumulative frequency distribution, *see* Frequency distribution, cumulative
Cut-off points, 18–19, 27

Data, 1, 9
  control, 55, 69, 106
  conversion of parametric to non-parametric, 2, 48, 107
  non-parametric, 1, 46
  paired, 54–55, 59, 73
  parametric, 2
    continuously variable, 9
    discontinuously variable, 9
  unpaired, 55, 70
Degrees of freedom, 75
  for analysis of variance, 86–87
  for χ^2, 38, 41, 42, 50, 92
  for correlation coefficient, r, 97, 102
  for F (variance ratio) tests, 71, 75
  for 't' tests, 75
    paired, 74
    unpaired, 73
  for 2 × 2 contingency tables, 51
Design, experimental, 3, 88, 106
Deviation, standard, *see* Standard deviation
Differences
  between means, 66–68, 70–76
  between proportions, 68–70
  see also Non-parametric tests of statistical significance; Tests of statistical significance
Distribution, 9
  binomial, 32–36, 42, 68–69
    approximation to normal, 33, 68
  chi-squared, *see* Chi-squared (χ^2)
  curves, 12, 13, 57, 71
  Gaussian, *see* normal

of means, 21–23
multinomial, 36
normal, 9, 12, 15, 22, 27, 39, 56, 85, 98, 107
  area under curve, 15–18, 27
  equation for curve, 12
Poisson, 36
skewed, 25–27, 28, 40, 107
  transformation to normal, 27, 40, 93

Error
  α error, see Type I
  β error, see Type II
  False positive, 19, 20
    see also Type I
  False negative, 19, 20
    see also Type II
  Type I, 5–6, 107
  Type II, 5–6, 48, 107
Error, standard, see Standard error
Expected value, 15
  of a mean difference, 73
Extrapolation
  from regression analysis, 101–102, 103

F-test for variances, 70–71, 78, 85, 87, 88
  see also Analysis of variance
Fisher's exact test, 52–53
Freedom, degrees of, see Degrees of freedom
Frequency distribution, 9, 13, 15
  absolute, 9–11
  cumulative, 9–11
  percentage, 9–11
Frequency polygon, 10

Goodness of fit to a hypothesis, 38, 39–41
Grouping data, 9, 38, 40, 59
Groups (columns), see Contingency tables, groups

Histogram, frequency, 9, 10, 11, 25
Hypotheses, 3–4, 108
  Alternative, 35
  Null, 4, 5, 34, 38, 48, 76–77, 107
    acceptance of, 6, 38
    rejection of, 6, 35
    testing, 4, 59, 78, 88

Incidence, 6
Independent variable, 95, 102
Intercept, 98, 99, 102

Linear regression, see Regression analysis
Logarithmic transformation, 27, 28, 41, 93, 99

Mann–Whitney test, see Wilcoxon's ranking test for unpaired data.
Mean, 12, 27, 95
  population, μ, 12, 13, 16, 21, 24, 66, 78, 85
    sample mean, comparison with, 21–24, 33, 66–67, 78
  sample, ($\bar{x}$), 12–13, 15, 16, 21, 66, 67–68, 70–73, 75–76, 78, 85
  standard error of, 21–24, 32, 66, 67, 70, 72
Measurement,
  non-parametric, scales of, 1
    nominal, 1
    ordinal (ranking), 1–2
  parametric, scale of, 2
    interval, 2
  transformations, 2
Median, 10, 11, 26, 27, 28
Modal group, 12, 13, 26, 27, 28

Non-parametric tests of statistical significance, 46, 56, 71, 107
  Chi-squared (χ^2), 47–52, 59
  Fisher's exact test, 52–53, 59
  sign test, 46–47, 59
  Spearman's rank correlation coefficient (ρ), 93–94, 102, 107
  Wilcoxon's ranking test for unpaired data, 55–58, 59–60
    z test for $n > 14$, 19, 57–58, 59
  Wilcoxon's signed rank test, 54–55, 59
Normal distribution, see Distribution, normal
Null hypothesis, see Hypothesis, Null

Observed value, 15, 91
  of a mean difference, 73
One-tailed test, 53, 76–77, 78
Outliers, 15, 27, 108

Partial correlation, 97
Population, 3, 13
  mean compared with sample, 66–67
Precision, 3
Predictive value, 19–21, 108
Prevalence, 6
  point, 6
  period, 6

Probability, 4–5, 16–18, 24, 52–53, 56, 70, 107

Quartiles, upper and lower, 10, 11, 27

Random sampling, 3, 32
Ranking, 2, 46, 54, 56, 59, 93
Rates, 6
  crude, 6–7
  standardized, 6–7
  survival, 11
Regression analysis, 95, 98–101, 102–103
  assumptions, 98
  curvilinear, 95, 98
  intercept, 98, 99, 102
  line of best fit, 94, 99–100, 102
  linear, 95, 98
  regression coefficient (slope), 98, 99, 102
    standard error of, 101, 102
    test for significance of, 101
Reliability, 3
Response (dependent) variable, 98
Rows, see Contingency tables, rows

Samples, 3
  bias in, 3
  paired, 54–55, 59
  random, 3, 32
  representative of population, 3, 32–33, 46
  selection of, 3, 106
  size, 3, 13, 15, 23, 28, 33, 42, 106
    large, 6, 15, 24, 33, 48, 66–70
    small, 6, 13, 15, 21, 23, 48, 70–76
  unpaired, 55
Scales of measurement, 1
  nominal, 1
  ordinal (ranking), 1–2
  interval, 2, 94
Scattergrams, 94, 95, 98, 102
Sensitivity, 20, 28, 108
Sign test, 46–47, 59
  comparison with signed rank test, 61
Significance, 5, 46, 59
  biological, 5, 91, 108
  statistical, 5, 6, 34, 59, 91, 108
  tests of, see Non-parametric tests of statistical significance; Tests of statistical significance
Skewed distribution of data, see Distribution, skewed
Slope, (regression coefficient), 98, 99–101, 102

Spearman's rank correlation coefficient (ρ), 93–94 102
Specificity, 20, 28, 108
Standard deviation, 12, 13–15, 16–17, 27
  about a regression line, 100
  combined (s_c), 71
  of p (s_p), 32–33
  population, 12, 14, 16, 85
  sample, 14, 85
Standard error, 21–24, 28, 32, 66
  combined, (SE_c), 68, 85
  of b, (SE_b), 101, 103
  of a mean difference, 67, 73
Standard normal deviate, z, 15–19, 27, 57, 66–70, 107
  z-test
    for assessing the significance of the regression coefficient, 101
    for comparing sample ($n > 30$) and population means, 66–67, 78
    for comparing two large ($n > 30$) sample means, 67–68, 78
    for comparing two percentages (both $n > 30$), 68–70, 78
    for small samples, F significant, 75, 78
    for Wilcoxon's ranking test, $n > 14$, 19, 57–58
Statistics, 1, 3
  choice of techniques, 106
  comparative, 4, 12, 46
  descriptive, 4, 12, 26, 46
Student's 't' test, 70
  degrees of freedom, 73, 74, 75, 78, 87, 101
  following analysis of variance, 87
  for significance of regression coefficient, 101, 103
  paired, 73–75, 78
  unpaired, 70–73, 78
Sum of squares, 14, 86, 88, 95
  between group, 86
total, 86
  within group (residual), 86

't' tests, see Student's 't' test
Tails of distribution curves, 15–16, 26, 58, 77
  see also One-tailed test; Two-tailed test
Tests of statistical significance
  comparison of parametric and non-parametric, 73, 74, 81–82
  comparison of 2 percentages, 68–70, 78

comparison of sample and
  population means, 66–67, 78
F-test, *see* F-test for variances
large samples, 66–70, 78
non-parametric, *see* Non-parametric
  tests of statistical significance
one-tailed, 53, 76–77, 78
small samples, 70–76, 78
  unpaired data, 70–73, 75, 78
  paired data, 73–75, 78
  F significant, 71, 75–76, 78
Student's 't' test, *see* Student's 't' test
two-tailed, 53, 68, 76–77, 78
Transformation of data, 27, 28, 93, 99
Two-tailed test, 53, 68, 76–77, 78
2 × 2 tables, 51–52, 59
  see also Contingency tables
Type I error, 5–6, 107
Type II error, 5–6, 48, 107

U (Mann–Whitney) test, *see*
  Wilcoxon's ranking test for
  unpaired data

Validity, 3
Variables,

continuous, 9
  dependent, 95, 102
  discontinuous, 9
  independent, 95, 102
  inter-related, 97
Variance, 13–15, 27, 69, 70–71, 78
  about a regression line, 100, 101, 103
  analysis of, *see* Analysis of variance
  between group, 85–88
  combined, 70
  comparison of 2, 70
    see also F-test for variances
  within group, 85–88
Variance ratio, *see* F-test for variances

Wilcoxon's ranking test for unpaired
  data, 55–58, 59–60
  z-test for $n > 14$, 19, 57–58, 60
Wilcoxon's signed rank test, 54–55, 59

Yates' correction for continuity, *see*
  Chi-squared (χ^2), Yates'
  correction

z, *see* Standard normal deviate